For Scott –

4/16/94
Seattle

BEYOND
RESULTS

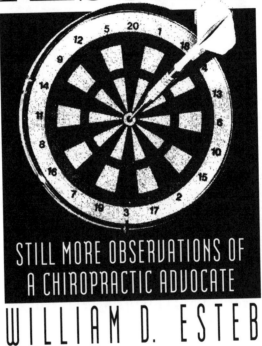

STILL MORE OBSERVATIONS OF
A CHIROPRACTIC ADVOCATE
WILLIAM D. ESTEB

P9-DEK-598

Published by Orion Associates

Also by William D.Esteb

A Patient's Point of View,
Observations of a Chiropractic Advocate

My Report of Findings,
More Observations of a Chiropractic Advocate

Published by
Orion Associates

Distributed by
Back Talk Systems, Inc.
2845 Ore Mill Drive, Suite 4
Colorado Springs, CO 80904-3161
(719) 633-1105 (800) 937-3113

Copyright (C) 1994 by William D. Esteb
All rights reserved including the right of reproduction
in whole or in part in any form.

Cover design by Buffalo Brothers, Inc.
Manufactured in the United States of America

Esteb, William D., 1952 -

Beyond Results
Still More Observations of a Chiropractic Advocate
ISBN 0-9631711-2-7

For Marilyn Gale Esteb

TABLE OF CONTENTS

FOREWORD

The camp is tense, there is a feeling of uncertainty in the air, everywhere you look there is anxiety, mixed with bravado. We all seem to know something unusual is happening. Will this mean an "inconvenience" for our lifestyle" Or will this mean a "paradigm shift," as Thomas Kuhn would say?

Many of us in the business of advising chiropractors believe that we are in for some major changes in the way we conduct ourselves as health care providers. Many will resist the changes or refuse to recognize them. Life has been sweet, why change?

William Esteb, as a chiropractic advocate, is in a unique position to provide direction for the profession. He is on the inside, but is still an outsider. He knows you. His writing and patient education aids show he also knows your patients. Although the advice is timeless, it is particularly useful to keep us on course during uncertainty.

Esteb has brought to chiropractic what Juran and Deming have brought to business management practice; a fresh viewpoint. Esteb has built a very convincing argument; things have changed. Drastically changed. The message is clear: adapt or die. The comforting part is the changes suggested will likely result in a personal sense of rightness, right action, greater self control and personal satisfaction.

He has written three books for us in the last few years. Each of the first two was justifiably well received, and addressed issues often skirted by other authors. This third one has done it again, in spades.

The future is bound to surprise us, but there is no need to be dumbfounded.

John T. Whitney, D.C.
Whitney Transition
Roswell, Georgia

1

INTRODUCTION

Want great results? Take ownership of these ideas and you'll get perpetually multiplying, omni-beneficial results. William D. Esteb is brilliant, insightful, eloquent, articulate, and offers chiropractors instantly useful ideas. I love, respect, admire, and appreciate this great man. His thinking and writing will influence chiropractic into the 21st century.

Esteb is the chiropractor's metaphorologist. A great metaphor states that the wine drank like liquid silk. Bill's writing is like liquid silk. It invites, provokes, captivates and creates new spaces of possibility.

Bill is a verbal artist painting a provocative new picture of the chiropractic profession. He will help you wake up to tomorrow, instead of being stuck in yesterday. Many doctors are whispering about memories of yesteryear. Bill wisely teaches that tomorrow is where the action is. Let's create it to be lavishly entreating, magnificently enticing, and omni-interesting. The future is the outpicturing of our current ideas.

I invite you to allow him to gently take your hand, guide your mind, and uplift your spirit to become all you can be in chiropractic and in life. Enjoy reading, digesting, and pondering my result-stimulating friend, William D. Esteb.

Mark Victor Hansen
Author of *Chicken Soup for the Soul* and *Dare to Win*
Newport Beach, California

SPECIAL THANKS

While only my name appears on the cover, I received a lot of help. Without the feedback and encouragement from countless doctors and staff members who have made me feel welcome in this profession, this book would not have been written.

Doctors who have been particularly instrumental include Claudia Anrig Howe, D.C., James Bowman, D.C., Robert DeMaria, D.C., Jeffry Finnigan, D.C., John Madeira, D.C., James Milliron, D.C., Tom O'Bryan, D.C., Elliott Segal, D.C., Greg Shaw, D.C., Lawrence Stern, D.C., Keith Thomson, D.C., Will Tickel, D.C., and the many others who called, asked questions at seminars, and generally forced me to clarify my ideas.

Others who have been influential over the years are Patricia Fox, Greg Stanley, Paul Franklin, Alan Lunsford, Bill Morr, Ed Edmunds, Andrea Ramsauer, and especially my Dad, Leonard Esteb, who taught and demonstrated the discipline and attention-to-detail that serves me today.

Special thanks to Robert D. Jackson, D.C., you are a wonderful friend and partner. And the entire Back Talk Systems, Inc. team, Debbie Richardson, Dusty Sorrentino, Sam and Robert Dick, Sharon Griffith, and Megan Kottwitz. Thanks for helping make what we do look so easy.

William D. Esteb
Colorado Springs, Colorado

THE NEW, NEW PATIENT

Like many other types of licensed professionals, getting new patients (clients, patrons, customers) is one of the most frequently mentioned concerns of today's chiropractor. This fixation has generated seminars, management programs, and advertising gimmicks designed to fill this perceived need. Unfortunately, the success of all too many of these programs are dependent upon a certain type of personality or manipulative communication techniques that make the typical doctor uncomfortable. Doctors who trust their own judgment and resist these approaches are accused of having a "poverty complex" or an "unwillingness to confront."

Those more sensitive to the dynamics of their discomfort recognize that the reason for their rejection of these techniques is that they realize that many times these new patient acquisition approaches do not honor the patient. New patients are often exploited, and treated in ways counter to the golden rule (treat others as you would have them treat you). The result is often a sense of frustration and impotence that can sabotage a doctor's self-worth enough to make the need for more patients even more acute!

The fact is, today's new patient is very different from the typical new patient showing up in chiropractic offices just five or six years ago. This change necessitates new approaches in the getting and keeping of new patients. Ignoring these trends, or continuing to d or say things counter to them, can result in a slow erosion of the number of new patients that show up on your doorstep.

Here are some of the major changes being seen among today's new patients:

The baby boomer: More and more of today's new patients were born between 1946 and 1964. The baby boom population in the United States is estimated at about seventy six million. They exert a tremendous influence on our culture today, and as they age, in this country's future. Weaned on the medical model of health, and lacking basic information in proper spinal hygiene, these patients are now showing up in chiropractic offices. A more complete exploration of their attitudes about health are covered in Ken Dychtwald's book, *Age Wave*.

Resistant to authority: More and more of today's new patients are the same college students who, when they weren't protesting the Viet Nam war, Dow Chemical, or ROTC recruitment policies, drove around college campuses with bumper stickers on the back of their VW Microbus that read, QUESTION AUTHORITY. And while much of this dogma has been tamed as they've married, had children, and entered mainstream society, many retain a certain amount of anti-establishment perspective. In fact, rebelling against medical authority figures with out of date communication skills is one of the reasons they're consulting chiropractors and other "alternative" providers! Their high level of education (more than 25% have college degrees) make them less susceptible to mindlessly following "doctor's orders" like their parents did. This is the generation that is increasingly seeking second opinions and echoing the same question their four-year olds are asking: why? More and more of today's new patients want to remain in control. The appropriate response? Adopt ' patient management style and abandon approach made popular in the 1980s.

Honor the patients' right and responsibility to make decisions about his or her health–even if it's not the wisest choice.

Visually oriented: Today's new patient is likely a member of the first TV generation, growing up with *Howdy Doody, Captain Kangaroo,* and *Sesame Street* and the countless dramas that took place in a medical setting (*Ben Casey, Dr. Kildare, Marcus Welby, M.D.,* etc.). Today's new patient is accustomed to having information spoon-fed by effortlessly watching TV. When patients are given the typical office brochure that requires lots of reading, it's just too much work.

Worse, many chiropractors are still giving reports of findings that are primarily oral presentations. For the previous generation that grew up listening to the radio and the soothing sounds of FDR's fireside chats, this approach worked fine. Today, the most effective communicators use pictures. Patients aren't racing home to get their hands dirty reading the newspaper. They channel surf the television, grazing for news.

Seek instant gratification: This is the generation that has grown up with instant coffee, microwave ovens, drive up windows, fast-acting sinus decongestion drugs, Federal Express, and FAX machines. Chiropractic, with its multiple-visit-long-term maintenance care orientation runs counter to this time-consciousness. You must change a patient's medically-taught one visit expectations. Their accelerated sense of time affects their tolerance for your withholding examination results until the formal report of findings, and even how long they'll have to wait in the reception room on subsequent visits. Many patients feel their time is just as valuable as the doctor's.

Assume a posture that suggests a reluctance to accept their case until they acknowledge that their problems didn't start last week when they "turned funny." Change their expectations. Explain the healing process. Reorient them by making comparisons to the process of mending a broken arm or the time it takes braces to affect structural changes with constant pressure. Make sure they don't buy into the "quick fix" mentality that directs much of the rest of their activities.

Image conscious: This is the generation that pays extra for brand name jeans, waits in line for Mazda Miatas, and subscribes to *Consumer Reports*. This concern with quality and image may thwart an inclination to consult an "alternative-non-mainstream-cult" form of healing like chiropractic. Chiropractic may not be high-tech enough. Chiropractic may be too vitalistic and philosophical for a generation that was taught that science holds all the answers.

Besides prompting patients to avoid chiropractic, the lack of a positive public image causes many patients, even those who get great results, from telling others about their chiropractic experiences. This resulting "chiropractic underground" is one reason why some of your best patients don't refer others. They'd prefer that no one knew they consulted a charismatic-free-spinal-exam-insurance-scam natural healer.

Make sure your bulletin boards and newsletters continue to include the results of recent research affirming chiropractic. Uncover each patient's fears and misconceptions and help them to be better equipped to defend their chiropractic decision to others. Ask patients what they've heard about chiropractic on their first visit.

Wellness outlook: This may be the most ironic trend of all. More and more of today's new patients have a wellness/preventive approach to their health. Beef consumption is down while that of fish and poultry is up. Distilled alcohol is down, beer (even nonalcoholic beer) and wine is up. Health clubs, high tech running shoes, exercise videos, and TV infomercials about the benefits of juicing, are part of the popular culture. This is good news for chiropractic because of its wellness orientation. But conventional wisdom suggests that chiropractic is only for bad backs! This perception has further distanced chiropractic from today's prospective new patient and the result of worshiping at the insurance alter during the 1980s. To gain "acceptance" (and cash-in on all the insurance money), all too many chiropractic offices have turned into pain relief clinics, even using the phrase "pain relief" in the office name!

Start emphasizing the wellness aspects of chiropractic care. Explain why *you* still get checked at least "X" number of times a month. Discuss why so many children receive care in your office. Explore the issues of subluxation degeneration and the non-symptomatic aspects of soft tissue damage that set the stage for relapse. Help your patients focus on how well they function, not just how well they feel.

More acute: On top of all these attitudes, today's new patients are more desperate when they arrive at your office. With fewer insurance policies having generously low deductibles, many patients wait until they can wait no longer before taking the plunge. Either because they are reluctant to submit to surgery, want to avoid being dependent upon drugs, refuse to "live with it," or are unwilling to pay for a second opinion, today's patients are waiting until the last minute before seeking care. The resulting personality distortion and compliance can fool you. During the early stages of their care they are quite compliant. Take advantage of their powerlessness and their compliance is often through unseen gritted teeth. Later, when they feel better they dismiss themselves, resenting the lack of respect they received during the earlier stages of care!

However the most obvious issue is financial. If the only type of insurance that most people can afford is catastrophic insurance (cancer, heart disease, etc.) with high deductibles, the cash practice is just around the corner. Even if these patients are inclined to refer others, their friends suffer from the same lack of financial assistance. The point? Wake up and smell the coffee! Get out of debt. Lower your overhead. Start weaning yourself from the upper reaches of what you extract from insurance companies. Seriously contemplate rejecting the notion of accepting assignment. Visualize your practice in the future when chiropractic may be more modestly priced without the assistance of the sickness care insurance industry.

Today's new patients are different than the generation just before them. Using old fashioned approaches to attract, communicate, and treat them in your office, is a prescription for frustration. ■

HOW TO PICK A
REAL CHIROPRACTOR

As I meet people outside the chiropractic profession and reveal my involvement in chiropractic, I am often asked, "How do you pick a good chiropractor?" Having been under care myself since 1981 and seen by five different doctors and adjusted by countless others, you might be interested in the criteria I give those preparing to investigate chiropractic.

Many of the people I talk to are suffering at the moment, brandishing a back brace, cervical collar, or massaging their necks. I suspect many are unhappy with their current treatment, or suspect chiropractic could help them but may have been disappointed with a previous brush with the profession. The horror stories they tell! Almost all the incidents revolve around a misunderstanding or lack of communication. Some expectation or unexpressed need wasn't addressed. The result is a disgruntled patient that vows never to return. Yet, they wonder if a different chiropractor could help, "I just don't want to go through the same thing I did with Dr. SoAndSo."

Each of the five doctors my family and I have been under care with are excellent doctors. I would, and have, recommended friends and family to each of them. And while many doctors often think the rejection by a patient is due to a technical flaw or a poor report of findings, that's rarely the case. I left one office because I didn't like smelling cigarette smoke on the doctor's clothing. We left another because the doctor didn't seem interested in creating a place where our three-year old would feel welcome. We left another because the affordable wellness care fees we were paying were suddenly eliminated. Still another took upwards of an hour to give a 4 minute adjustment. While some delivered better adjustments than others, they were all excellent.

As I think back over the years, one thing does seem significant. Each doctor eventually assumed an attitude that I would remain a patient for the rest of my life. I had become part of the expected "office volume." I was being taken for granted. Like any customer, when the business establishment doesn't acknowledge or show their appreciation for repeat business or continued patronage, it's easy to justify a change in one's purchasing habits.

"It's always good to see you," smiles the doctor. "I always look forward to the days I see your name on the appointment book," beams the front desk assistant. "How can we continue to make your visits with us more enjoyable?" asks the doctor between notations on the patient's travel card. "What's the favorite part of your visit with us?" wonders a staff person outloud. Make observations or ask questions that communicate your continuing interest and appreciation in the patient. Only this type of display of conscious caring can transcend the when-the-symptoms-are-gone-I'm-through-with-chiropractic attitude that many patients have. Everyone wants to feel wanted and appreciated. Especially people who have to dig into their own pocket to pay for their care!

Another observation. Not once since 1981, have I received a formal progressive examination and report. Coincidence, or is this lack of continued accountability rampant in the profession? Seems to me, a regular examination every twelve visits or so, could help keep the patient *and* the doctor focused on the job at hand. Offices that were "new patient machines" in the early 1980s could afford to let patients fade away because more new patients with low insurance deductibles were waiting in the wings. Making patients feel continually welcome and appreciated, while affirming their decision to be in your office, is essential these days. Especially with so many of their friends ready to judge their mental faculties for consulting a chiropractor in the first place!

"But at some point, there isn't any measurable improvement in their examination findings," I can almost hear you say.

That's right. Isn't the first objective to get patients feeling better and the second to maximize complete healing and function? Congratulations! Now the patient is ready for the type of chiropractic care you and your veteran staff members enjoy: wellness care. Why do you continue to receive adjustments? Be sure to reveal your personal care program to your patients. Explain why *you* continue to get adjusted and why *you* expect to receive care for the rest of your life. Remember, you're setting an example with everything you say and do.

With what I know today, here are a few guidelines I'd use to find a new chiropractor or advice I'd give someone considering beginning care. Would your office qualify?

1. Is the office near where you live or work? You can't do to much about this one except recognize that for the most part there is a "farming" area for new patients. Yes, there is the rare doctor with the special something extra that can prompt patients to drive miles for an adjustment. For the average doctor, get a detailed map of your area and draw a circle around a three to five mile radius. What's there? Homes or businesses? Blue collar or white collar? High income or low? Do the kinds of patients you enjoy spending time with live in your area?

2. Do they offer a no obligation visit? I'm not talking about a free spinal exam! What I'm talking about is, does the office solicit prospective patients to tour the office, meet and interview the doctor, and get questions asked without cost or obligation? Does the office recognize the myths and misconceptions today's patient brings with him or her to the office and offer ways to "ease into" this new relationship?

3. Can I talk to other patients with the same problem I have? I can't figure out why more offices don't do this. As patients show improvement, ask them if they'd be willing to sign up for your Nervous New Patient Program. What's that? "Sometimes we have people call us up to begin care and we can tell they're somewhat nervous. So we ask some of our regular patients if they wouldn't mind fielding occasional phone calls from prospective new patients. That way, patients with headaches (or low back pain or whatever) can ask questions and have a lot of their concerns addressed by an experienced chiropractic veteran like you." The testimonial book out in the reception room doesn't fill this need. A nervous patient would want to interview your veteran patients and ask specific questions *before* showing up in your office.

4. What type of patient education do they offer? This reveals a lot. If the office merely gives a report of findings and expects patients to help themselves to a brochure rack of 1962 health tracts, I counsel my friends to keep looking. The amount of systematic patient education is a good indication of the doctor's chiropractic philosophy, emphasis on patient responsibility, and commitment to long term rehabilitative and wellness care. Of course there are brochures, but do they give lectures, use videos, or other technologies to consistently communicate chiropractic? Offices with a strong commitment to patient education, (also revealed by a well-trained staff that can answer questions), are most likely going to offer new patients an excellent chiropractic experience. Offices that overlook patient education keep patients in the dark, making it easier to control them. Poor patient education often means a "pain clinic" atmosphere that shortchanges the patient and their health.

5. Do they take X-rays? I've heard all the arguments for and against this issue and personally I'd be a little nervous if the doctor didn't take X-rays. That doesn't' mean that every seven-year old should routinely get a Davis series! What I'm interested in, is whether the doctor is sensitive to a biomechanical model of the spine? Does he or she take post X-rays and recognize that functional changes can be, and should be, expected from appropriate chiropractic care?

6. Do they see very many children? Lots of children in the practice (10% of office visits or more) is a good sign. It confirms there is good patient education and suggests parents trust the doctor. Any chiropractor who can build rapport with a child has my vote for being able to build rapport with an adult. It doesn't always work the other way! Also, having a lot of children in the office tells me about the doctor's adjusting skills (excellent), his or her office environment (stimulating), and communication skills (effective).

7. Do they regularly give (and get) referrals to the medical community? Knowing when to refer out is an important diagnostic skill the best chiropractors posses. The macho I-can-handle-anything-that-walks-or-crawls-through-the-door attitude is out of touch, egotistical, and frankly dangerous. Knowing one's limits is a sign of maturity. Give chiropractic a chance, but rise above the bigotry and bias. Avoid turning the patient into a pawn in some old fashioned battle with the medical community. The reverse is true, too. Do medical doctors feel comfortable enough with the office to entrust their patients with a chiropractor?

Notice that none of the probing questions I recommend has anything to do with what school you graduated from, your age, adjusting technique, politics, or philosophy! Funny how the issues that get the pulse quickening among doctors has little to do with the criteria *patients* use to select a good doctor. Funny how yellow page ads rarely address issues that prospective patients are interested in. Funny how many offices put the newest, least experienced staff member at the front desk to field these questions. Funny. Ha-ha. ■

A NEW PATIENT'S GREATEST CONCERNS

While there is a fixation on new patients in this profession, it's easy for the doctor and staff to forget what a new patient is going through. Remember that their symptoms distort their personalities. Their fears of the unknown impede cooperation in subtle ways. Their misconceptions about chiropractic interfere with rapport. Their expectations are based on a lifetime of indoctrination by visits to medical providers. Ignoring these issues, because patients aren't bold or assertive enough to raise them, invites misunderstandings and poor compliance.

Except in the most disorganized offices, new patient procedures are routine. The doctor and staff are well acquainted with the new patient admitting form that is presented, yet this is the first time the patient has ever seen it. The first visit protocol is well practiced and automatic for the staff and doctor, yet everything is new to the patient. In short, the office and procedures are familiar and second nature to those who work in it every day. But to the patient they can be intimidating and anxiety producing. Fooled by the lack of questions from the patient, it is easy to breeze through those initial visits without bringing the patient into the inner circle and getting them involved in their care.

Today's patients bring with them, a set of unspoken concerns about what they are going to encounter in your office. Recognizing and acknowledging these concerns, while creating communication strategies to put patients at ease, promotes respect and raises the patients' self esteem. Patients work hard to cover up their feelings of being alone and frightened.

Here are some common concerns patients bring with them on their first visit or two, plus some approaches you might want to consider to reduce their defensive postures and enhance the healing process:

"Is it going to hurt?" Conventional wisdom tells patients that if a particular spinal joint hurts when they enter your office, working with the joint is going to hurt even more. In fact, it is often this misguided notion that chiropractic care is painful, that delays many patients from seeking care. Yet, the painful symptoms often result in total compliance with every doctor request. Others, who grasp at anything to maintain their dignity and remain in control, may make light of the adjustment or "crack" jokes about the procedure. Still others are praying so loudly you might actually hear them while giving them their first adjustment!

Action step: Some doctors take a few moments before rendering the first adjustment to discuss their adjusting approach, "Think of an adjustment as lifting a heavy weight off your toe." Considering mentioning that, as of the last count, this new patient is about to receive somewhere in the vicinity of your 250,000th adjustment, or whatever the number might be. Let your new patient know that your adjustments are precise and you are well experienced in giving them. This is one area in which older, more experienced doctors have a perceived advantage over the new doctor.

"Do I have to take off my clothes?" Even in the 1990s this is still a concern among many new patients. Again, rarely spoken, it can be the underlying cause of a resistance to an X-ray examination or even consulting your office!

Action step: Besides mentioning the extent to which new patients will need to disrobe at the beginning of your examination, consider adding locks to the door of the room in which you'll be asking them to change in. Also, instead of the demeaning, open back gowns used in hospitals, look at the possible use of surgical scrubs or two-piece jogging suit for X-ray procedures. Even if patients don't seem concerned, demonstrate your respect for their privacy by implementing procedures and orienting your office environment to the most modest patients.

"Will I have to come for the rest of my life?" This is a bigger concern than many doctors realize. The challenge here is that the hidden, or not so hidden agenda of most offices is to collect chiropractic clients that adopt a preventive/maintenance visit schedule for the rest of their lives. Yet, during the first visits, you have not yet earned the right to even suggest this type of chiropractic lifestyle. First you must prove you can help them with the problem they've presented to you. In the same way an increasing number of patients wish to avoid being dependent upon aspirin, pain pills, or muscle relaxers, they don't want to be dependent on a doctor prescribing regular adjustments! Ironically, successfully addressing and overcoming this independence issue is important if you want more cash-paying maintenance patients in your practice.

Action step: Reassure new patients that they are in the right place by acknowledging that your first responsibility is to help them with their presenting health compliant. Use the likely success with their problem as a way of earning the right to talk about a bigger vision of chiropractic for their optimum health. During your report of findings give an overview of the realistic amount of time (visits) likely needed to heal and maintain their condition, yet package your recommendations in bite-sized periods of a dozen visits or so. Patient education is critical during this initial stage of care. Explain to patients how your *own* family is receiving care, and how frequently you continue to receive adjustments, even though you're not obviously symptomatic. Assuming this mentor role may be new to you, but it is essential.

"Can I afford this?" Today, with financial policies and insurance coverage in flux, this is perhaps one of the most important concerns the most responsible patients have. Interestingly, chiropractic is one of the few licensed professional services in which doctors seem able to separate some pie-in-the-sky treatment plan, from what it actually costs a patient. Doctors seem uncomfortable telling patients what the cost of their care will be. "When we're finished here, Barbara will go over what all this is going to cost." And while most doctors don't delegate enough routine office procedures to their staff, this is one area most doctors need to rethink.

Perhaps doctors (who get their care free) can separate the treatment plan from its cost, but patients don't. So while doctors outline a grand treatment schedule and the benefits of optimum spinal function, patients are distracted by trying to multiply the number of recommended visits by the cost per visit. What many doctors overlook is that most patients walk into the office with a figure in their mind as to how much they think their problem should cost to get fixed. "It's going to cost how much?" roars the skeptical spouse when your new patient returns home with the news. If a patient walks in thinking their problem is worth about $350 to correct, you have two choices. One, is to have such a high entry fee for your examination and X-rays that a large portion of that $350 is used up before any kind of treatment is rendered, or, lower your entry fee so they can afford enough visits to see some progress before running out of money! It's up to you.

Action steps: While few patients will reveal the amount of money they have tentatively reserved for chiropractic care, recognize that they probably have one. (Patients with higher self-esteem and income probably have a higher figure.) Reevaluate your entry fees based on this reality. Create a menu of different financial programs to help patients find one that works for them. Begin discussing the financial implications of your care recommendations. Analyze your fee schedule and determine if it still makes sense in light of fewer and fewer patients even having insurance.

"What will my friends think?" Peer pressure and "what will my neighbors think" are still major factors that influence how people act in our society. It takes a brave soul to go against the "accepted" and the "approved" to consult an alternative, non-mainstream form

of health care. Besides making the new patient feel even more alone, it can thwart the referral process. The resulting "chiropractic underground" continues to slow the acceptance of chiropractic among a generation in search of what's hot and what's not. For many, chiropractic isn't "correct" enough. Yet.

Action steps: Equip patients with information that overcomes common myths and misconceptions about chiropractic. Make sure they know your educational achievements, training, why drugs aren't used, the safety of adjustments, why you chose chiropractic over medicine, and address the other myths and misconceptions still plaguing much of the general public. Make certain that your current patients have the ammunition to defend their chiropractic decision, so they will more likely divulge their chiropractic experience with others.

Chiropractic, even with the recent advancements, will continue to depend upon the inclination of current patients to tell others. Waiting for the drug-controlled media or your state association fund raising efforts to implement needed public relations programs, is likely going to be a long wait. Make sure the relief your patients experience from your skillful hands is duplicated by the psychological relief of having their fears and concerns addressed. ■

WHAT PATIENTS EXPECT

When a new patient enters your practice, besides a headache or low back pain, they bring with them a set of expectations. These expectations have been created by their experiences with other health care providers, the media, the opinions of their friends and family, and are exaggerated by feelings of pain, fear, and sometimes hopelessness. Ignore these expectations and you risk being perceived as an insensitive mechanic. Merely meet these expectations and you have a satisfied patient. Exceed these expectations and you have a delighted, enthusiastic patient with reasons to tell others about their experience in your office. Do you know what your patients' expectations are?

Ironically, successfully meeting and exceeding patient expectations starts with your staff. How the doctor treats the staff is the guideline the staff uses to treat patients. If staff members are kept in the dark about office goals, long term objectives, changes in office policy, so are patients. If staff members are kept guessing as to the doctor's expectations of them, staff members are less likely to make apprehensive patients comfortable by volunteering information to patients about what to expect. If the doctor doesn't make an emotional investment in the staff, the staff is unlikely to make an emotional investment in the patients, making them feel like outsiders rather than practice "members." Uncovering and responding to patient expectations is intrinsically a leadership issue.

Because of the inbreeding found in chiropractic (and most other professions), many of the expectations doctors think new patients have, are outdated. Worse, many doctors are totally unaware of many new patient expectations. If ignored, these unmet expectations create a "moving target" that hampers efforts to satisfy patients and create optimum new patient rapport. Overlooking a patient's expectations is expensive.

How do you uncover your patient's expectations? Ask. Rarely do new patients enter your practice with a written list of their first visit questions. Few patients are bold or assertive enough to grill you about your policies or procedures. Don't think that their silence means they're not interested or they're willing to automatically comply! What their personality distorting physical symptoms, combined with their socially-induced low self-esteem are saying, is that the fear of the unknown has been eclipsed by a throbbing headache, an inability to turn their heads, or the alarming numbness in their legs.

If their curiosity isn't enough to prompt them to ask questions, and the doctor or staff neglect to volunteer information, patients never feel included and remain distant and detached. Being open with patients, anticipating their concerns, and helping create a forum where they can safely discuss their needs, is comforting and affirming. To do so projects an attractive form of clinical self-confidence that draws patients in and makes them feel welcome.

What are typical new patient first visit expectations? Of course it varies, depending upon the patient's socio-economic background, educational achievements, and previous health care experiences. Here are some issues worth considering as you evaluate your first visit protocol in light of being more sensitive to your new patients' expectations:

Professional office setting: Like women in the corporate world who have to do their job twice as good to be considered equal to a man, chiropractic must project the contemporary, up-to-date image patients see in the highly-polished images of medicine on television. Because chiropractic is an intangible service, patients can't tell if their experience is going to be a good one until they submit to care, by walking in the front door of your office. Their first impression of your office location, size, and decor allude to the quality of care they suspect they will receive. A shabby reception room suggests shabby chiropractic care.

Relevant paperwork: Everyone knows there's paperwork to be completed when beginning a new relationship with a health care provider. Besides being brief and of high quality (no bad copies of bad copies of faint originals!), the paperwork must seem relevant to the reason(s) the patient has come to your office. Seemingly esoteric questions about whether they were delivered by forceps (who remembers?), were immunized (what does that have to do with my "slipped disc?"), or have some form of sexual dysfunction (it's none of your business!), should be asked privately by the doctor if they are truly relevant to the patient's case. From a patient's point of view, many of these questions are as relevant as asking for their astrological sign or whether the hospital they had their tonsils removed was Catholic or Protestant!

Honoring the appointment time: While more and more offices are abandoning appointment times for regular visits by established patients, setting specific appointments for first, second, and progress exam visits is probably still a good idea. As time becomes a more valuable commodity in our fast-paced-drive-up-window lifestyles, running on time communicates respect for the patient. Because this may be a new experience for most patients, be sure to volunteer how long you expect the first visit to take. Otherwise, patients can become testy, glancing at their watches, shifting in their seats, and looking at the door during your explanation of the three curves of the spine.

See other patients: Ever walk into a recommended restaurant at the height of the dinner hour only to find it practically empty? The same feeling can overcome new patients who walk into an empty reception room. Without an explanation that "...we've reserved some special time between our regular patients to get you started..." a new patient can reach the conclusion that they've consulted a less than successful practitioner. Cluster book as much as you can, bringing new patients into the office as close to your "rush hour" as you can adequately handle.

Interview the doctor: It sounds backwards to doctors, but patients want to "like" their doctor as much as respect him or her. The most discerning patients expect the doctor to reveal enough about him or herself so that they can determine if they respect the doctor. That doesn't mean you need to "sell" yourself or be a "buddy," but take the opportunity to personalize examples ("You have a problem much like mine...") or relate experiences you had during the early stages of your own care. The key is to break through the "doctorly" image that served to impress a previous generation, yet insulates you from today's patients who want reassurance that they've consulted a "real" person and not a fringe fanatic.

Privacy: It goes without saying that if you want patients to reveal their deepest, darkest, health care secrets, patients expect privacy. Do new patients hear the front desk staff talking about other patients (by name!) while waiting in the reception room? Make sure patients have every reason to trust you and your office before you ask them to divulge personal information.

Address financial issues: While many doctors recognize the importance of optimum spinal function and can somehow divorce the cost of care from the care itself, patients don't. Most patients walk into the office with some internal gauge as to how much their recovery should cost, or how much they're willing to spend on themselves. While most patients won't volunteer this figure (or admit they have one), it is the subtext of most doctor/patient conversations about the recommendations for care. This is the one psychological and financial advantage of having some type of case fee arrangement for the initial stages of pain relief. Patients, particularly the most responsible ones, expect the financial ramifications of their chiropractic commitment to be addressed.

Treatment on the first visit: You had better have a powerful argument for not treating the patient on their first visit! The medical community has taught patients that relief of their ache or pain is as close as enduring the office visit, getting the prescription, and ingesting the medicine. Ignore this fundamental expectation and you risk patient disappointment and even alienation. While delaying care, even holding their X-rays hostage until they attend a lecture, is an effective power ploy, most patients resent the abuse. Take the X-rays, look at the X-rays, and show them to the patient on a subsequent visit accompanied by a complete report of findings, but help the poor patient who has already indulged in your every command!

These common patient expectations, combined with the countless individual apprehensions every new patient has, are largely the result of a fear of the unknown. Imagine the result if this instant everyone in the country knew what happens on the first visit to a chiropractic office! Just about everyone knows what happens in a medical doctor's office or a dentist's office. It is this fear of the unknown, coupled with a set of preconceived notions, that serves as an effective barrier to an investigation of chiropractic. Instead, everyday, thousands of patients are opting for drastic measures such as surgery, artificial distortion of their immune systems, and countless other barbaric procedures, because they are afraid.

What are you doing (or not doing) because you're afraid? ∎

VALIDATING THE PATIENT

It's easy to forget how dependent and not-like-normal patients are when they come into your office. They've waited sometimes weeks, maybe months, before dialing the seven digits of your office phone. The person that shows up is not the real person, but a distant and rudimentary cousin. At any other time in this person's life they're cracking jokes and being the life of the party. When they show up in your office they're introspective, internal, and painfully aware of the decision they've just made: consulting a chiropractor. The last resort. The bottom of the barrel. The low man on the totem pole. Are they excited about "turning on the force" or dreaming about "their human potential?" Hardly. These poor patients need even more affirmation and validation than chiropractors! And what are they faced with? A new patient admitting form and a front desk assistant with the attitude of "business as usual." No wonder new patient rapport seems elusive and impossible. No wonder new patients don't "get it." No wonder patients discontinue care after symptomatic relief. No wonder!

Because we are trained to be "right" in our culture, and few new patients on their first couple of visits know if the decision to consult a chiropractor's office was "right," many new patients withhold approval and opt not to participate in what would be totally beneficial office procedures. Their reluctance and perceived skepticism is the direct result of not receiving sufficient validation for making the decision to consult your office. Ironically, the negativity and "prove it" attitude that doctors encounter with some patients is the direct result of not acknowledging the new patient and providing sufficient validation.

If we're hungry and sit down to a plate of pancakes and feel full 10 minutes later–that's validation. When we answer the *Jeopardy* question or solve the *Wheel of Fortune* puzzle before the on-camera contestants, we are validated. When we dazzle a friend by taking them to a new restaurant or movie they end up liking, we are validated. Validation comes from affirmation, exceeding the expectations of others, or the opportunity to show our good judgment or "rightness." To bad new chiropractic patients receive so little validation for their decision to consult your office! The validation, when it comes, can be weeks later when their symptoms finally subside. For the patients who drop out after a visit or two, that apparently isn't good enough!

Here are some ideas you may want to consider to help new patients feel more at home and validate their decision to consult your office:

1. Get testimonials. Funny how some of the old ideas are still the best. Are you collecting testimonials from your patients? Get started! There's nothing quite as reassuring as a "real" person without an axe to grind who talks up chiropractic. Ask your most articulate patients if they'd be available to field occasional phone calls from new patients who are especially apprehensive. Collect these patients' names and their comments in a three-ring binder. Organize it by primary complaint. Then you can recommend that anxious new patients call a patient who has had success with the same problem they have. Make it accessible to new patients in the reception room, too.

2. Honor the patient. There are many ways to honor patients (giving them more respect than they give themselves), but the easiest way is to let them know what's going to happen before it happens. It's so easy to get into your "new patient groove" and forget that this isn't the patient's 250th new patient experience–it's their first. Let them know what you're doing, and why, in advance of every procedure. Over-communicating in this way projects a sensitive and caring attitude that new patients appreciate. Remember, they're probably in pain, afraid of the unknown, and not their usual selves. Don't wait for questions. Volunteer the information.

3. See other patients like themselves. Those who cluster book already understand this phenomenon. New patients want to see others like themselves in your reception room. Scheduling new patients at slow times of the day may be handy for you, but it can be unsettling for the patient unless it is explained. You'd question your friend's restaurant recommendation if you showed up and it was virtually empty at the dinner hour. Same with patients. Streamline your office procedures so you can successfully accommodate new patients during the busy times of the day. New patients want assurance that they've picked a successful doctor.

4. Speak a language patients understand. This may be the most difficult. Ever try explaining chiropractic to an 8th grader? It requires abandoning the vocabulary you're accustomed to. Watch for the glazed-eye reaction to words like adjustment, subluxation, and interference, not to mention the MRI, IME, and other acronyms that can work their way into patient conversations if you're not careful. The objective isn't to talk down to a patient, just use words and metaphors that patients understand. If you want to use the big $50 words first, then explain them, fine. The key is to bring each patient into the "inner circle" of their care. That way chiropractic care isn't something that merely happens to them. What people don't understand, doesn't exist.

5. Care about patients beyond their expectations. Every management expert in the profession will tell you to avoid this one. The only problem is, the most successful offices get involved in the lives of their patients. Besides, how can you avoid it when you're working with the fundamental elements of life? Volunteer to help solve transportation problems, refer locksmiths, recommend interior designers, and direct patients to other resources that may have nothing to do with their health. Become a trusted resource for your patients. No need to become nosy—simply become a problem solver.

6. Increase the patient's self-esteem. That's what these validation suggestions really do. If patients always feel better about themselves mentally, socially, and spiritually by being around you, guess what your patients will want to do? Of course! "Oh, you look so good in blue." "It's great that you're always on time for your appointments." "I saw a wonderful book yesterday and I immediately thought of you." The list goes on and on. The point is to be conscious enough to see the individual beauty of every patient. Remember, all too many of your patients have endured a life of being ignored, put down, manipulated, and abused. Offer them the affirmation that automatically comes when you stop seeing them as part of your day's volume, but as the individuals that they really are.

Notice that few of these suggestions have little to do with the therapeutics of chiropractic. Chiropractic is merely the "entry point" or the opportunity that brings patients into contact with you. The fact that they have low back pain or headaches and consult your office is merely the practical reason for needing you. The intangible qualities of validation, esteem, rapport, and affirmation can decide if your relationship will be a brief encounter or a life long friendship. The most fulfilling arrangement is a long term connection. It is the forum for the most rewarding kinds of healing and the kind of affirmation you deserve. An endless stream of sick patients that you repeatedly get well, so you can prove to yourself that chiropractic works, becomes old quickly. It is the fodder of burnout. The real joy in chiropractic is when you look forward to coming to your office because you are surrounded by friends, which happens to be the same joy *patients* want to feel when they come to your office. ■

JUSTIFYING DECISIONS

In another era of my life I dated a woman who enjoyed old, romantic, black and white movies. The ones with Betty Davis, Fred Astaire, Ginger Rogers, and Gene Kelly. I'd watch her watch these movies, enchanted by the language, drama, costumes, and grass-growing plot development. If there was dancing, all the better. It was because I enjoyed *her*, not the movies she liked, that I reluctantly agreed to investigate ballroom dancing lessons.

After we found the place, and climbed up the stairs to the second floor, I began questioning my decision. The air smelled of stale cigarette smoke and the drab 15-year old hallway carpet was notice-ably worn. When we entered the dance studio we were greeted by a brightly-lit oak dance floor, surrounded by hundreds of mirrors. Several couples, 40 years our seniors, were on the floor dancing to the distorted, crackling music blaring from a portable stereo at the other end of the room. My girlfriend was instantly captivated. I was instantly uneasy about what I was getting myself into.

We were met by a plump and overly bejeweled woman in her 50s who began calling each of us "honey" as she led us to a side office off the dance floor. To make an embarrassing story as short as possible, I was suckered into signing up for an eight-week course costing close to $500. I didn't feel good about it as it was happening, and still didn't feel good about it on each of the subsequent Wednes-day evenings when I tried in vain to get my feet to do things Gene Kelly's did.

I had a bad "feeling" about the experience from the very beginning. I couldn't put my finger on it, but I resented the hard sell close, the "divide and conquer" sales technique, and the "buy now and save" attitude of desperateness she conveyed. I was committed to my girlfriend more than to the lessons. Frankly, I was there for the wrong reasons. About three lessons into the contract we broke up and I was able to extricate myself out of the lessons and the relationship.

Bert Decker, in his book, *You've Got To Be Believed To Be Heard*, suggests that each of us make decisions based upon how we feel, and later justify them with facts. How true. My problem with the dance lessons was I started out on the wrong foot (so to speak) by not "feeling" good about the decision, and didn't receive sufficient affirming facts and information (feedback) during the early stages of the lessons to solidify and justify my decision.

The same process happens in chiropractic.

Patients make their initial decision to consult your office based on a feeling. Patient education offers the facts on which to justify their decision to consult an alternative healer who is "unapproved" by their HMO or social group. Patient education helps avoid buyer's remorse. It solidifies the relationship and helps affirm the patient's decision to consult your office.

In my ballroom dancing lesson experience I didn't feel good about the situation and this prevented any deepening of the relationship through the transmission of information or facts. Decker is right. If people don't trust you, they don't hear what you have to say. This issue has been lost on those fixated on the right technique, the right report of findings script, or the right recall script. The words have little meaning if the patient doesn't fundamentally trust you. Improving this level of trust is possible, if you're interested. Yet, all too many doctors would prefer to ignore or overlook this issue. It's much more convenient to focus on other more concrete issues like adjusting technique, X-ray interpretation, multiple visit recommendations, and other things that are less vague or require less ambiguity in their implementation.

Successfully dealing with this "soft" aspect of patient relationships predicts a doctor's ability to build rapport and prevent patient misunderstandings and disappointments–critical issues to the referral process and the willingness of patients to comply with your recommendations. Again, this is why doctors with a well developed personality or a demonstrative, external, tableside manner are so successful. The sensitivity and ability to adapt and appropriately respond to each individual patient's need for reassurance is a key element. Instead, many of the best "technicians" limp along in their practices, thinking their clinical awards from school will make up for this shortcoming.

The key is to recognize this process and take a proactive role by affirming the "correct" decisions patients make, not only by beginning care in the first place, but continuing with care, referring their friends, and being responsible. Here are some specific action steps to consider:

Anticipate concerns. If you were a new patient who knew nothing about chiropractic, what would be some of your concerns? Brainstorm these topics with your staff. Then, develop a systematic way of anticipating these patient concerns and volunteering appropriate information in advance; "Right about now, many of our patients start wondering if..." "I always spend a few moments on each patient's third visit to share an observation..." Anticipating someone else's needs or concerns is perceived as extraordinary.

Ask questions. Ask open ended questions about the patients' perceptions about the direction, speed, and effectiveness of their care program. Not because you're defensive or lack conviction! Solicit feedback so you can personalize your patient education efforts. Patient education must be a dialogue, not a monologue; afferent/efferent. Waiting for patients to volunteer a comment or being surprised by their sudden lack of compliance, invites disappointment. Ask.

Stop the process. Remember, you're the one in charge. Don't use patient feedback as an opinion poll. Patients want leadership from their doctor. If you sense the patient misunderstands something or shows signs of disrespect for you or chiropractic, put the brakes on!

Discontinue the exam, the adjustment, or whatever. Own the idea that patients need you a whole lot more than you need them. Patients are guests, and guests don't insult the host or make fun of the host's career choice.

Involve the staff. Make sure the staff understands the dynamic of volunteering information to patients. Not just what is going to happen, but why. We tire quickly of unexplained waiting, procedures that don't make sense, and seemingly irrelevant questions. Volunteering why there is a delay, why cervical X-rays are being taken for a low back problem, why they have to gown, and all the other "whys" can serve to reassure the patient. Since staff members generally spend more time with the patient than the doctor, make sure they are qualified to volunteer information on these topics.

Provide patient referrals. With all information presented in the office, from either the doctor or the staff, patients expect to hear the "company line." Pure, unadulterated information is available from actual patients. But patients who still haven't yet made a commitment need help identifying patients they could ask questions about what really goes on. Refer hesitant new patients to "good" patients who have volunteered to field questions from apprehensive beginners.

How do your patients feel about continuing care on a nonsymptomatic basis? How do your patients feel about entrusting their children with you for care? How do your patients feel about paying for their care? How do your patients feel about their initial care requiring three visits a week? How do your patients feel about X-rays? Your financial policies? Therapy? Signing in? Without facts to back up the rationale for these concepts and procedures, they can seem arbitrary and gratuitous to patients. Reinforce the feelings of trust, affirm their decision to be in your office, and follow your recommendations. No need to be defensive! Be proactive, confident, and appreciate that your patient's previous experiences in a health care environment were probably very different from yours. Be proud of your difference and uniqueness. Just remember to explain why. ■

DO PATIENTS GET IT?

Clearly, the doctors who are the best communicators have the best practices. It's the only thing that can begin to explain why your college friends you helped through Organic Chemistry have large practices! Patients are buying you and your personality, not your grade point average. And while it's easy to sneer at high volume practitioners and convince yourself they must be providing slip-shod chiropractic care, doing something illegal, or both, this form of bigotry reveals more about you than the accused. Patients choose doctors and other professionals on *their* criteria–not yours. And for many patients, a doctor's openness and ability to project caring and confidence are more attractive than a long stream of initials after one's name. Unfortunately, personality may be more important than clinical excellence.

This doesn't negate the importance of good examination skills, adjusting technique, and superb record keeping. Naturally the symptomatic results patients seek in a chiropractic office must occur too. The glue that holds these technical issues together, along with the willingness to withhold judgment about chiropractic long enough to get the symptomatic relief they seek in your office, is the doctor's ability to communicate confidence and hope.

Certainly the simple skill of active listening is valuable here. So too, is the common sense and discipline necessary to avoid rushing in and spouting anti-medicine epitaphs and your chiropractic philosophy. *When* to say something is just as important as *what* you say. It means seeing situations in your office (that by now you take for granted) from a patient's point of view. It requires honoring the patient where they *are* so you can earn the right to take them where they need to go.

Honoring the patient means you actively look for opportunities to raise a patient's self-esteem. Honoring the patient means treating them with more respect than they treat themselves. Honoring the patient means anticipating their needs and concerns and volunteering information. Honoring the patient means that you still respect them when they make a poor decision. Honoring the patient acknowledges that the patient is always right–just not necessarily correct!

Notice that honoring the patient does not mean that you allow the patient to manipulate or exploit you or your staff. It does not mean that the patient has a free rein to dictate policy or procedure. Interestingly, offices that truly honor the patient rarely see anger or disrespect from their patients. When the office and its policies are consistent, fair, and affirm the patient's self-respect, they naturally create a healing environment that is attractive.

Regardless of your intent, if patients perceive that they are merely a number, dehumanized by a lack of privacy, or countless other more subtle oversights, it can set in motion various types of patient behavior. To doctors it can make patient conduct seem capricious or unexplainable.

Skepticism: Patients who enter your office and go through your procedures with their arms crossed, either physically or figuratively, are sending an important message. It's a defense mechanism that allows those who are self-conscious or resent their apparent lack of control in your domain to maintain their dignity. Careful! Skepticism may be an indication of their lack of respect or a way of holding onto their current, yet failed, model of health. It may merely mean a resistance to change. It's an important symptom, but don't take it personally.

Lack of responsibility: Patients who act irresponsible may be doing so because the doctor has assumed the hero roll. When the doctor accepts the role of health care savior, he or she usurps the patient's responsibility. Worse, few offices outline the specific patient responsibilities necessary to be accepted as a patient. "Unlike other types of health care, chiropractic is a partnership approach. You have some important responsibilities to fulfill if we are going to accept you as a new patient." When doctors or staff members project the attitude that they are overly anxious to accept anyone with a spine as a new patient, they send a message that may diminish the patient's willingness to take their care seriously.

Drop out: Yes, patients drop out because they get the symptomatic relief for which they originally consulted your office. Without patient education that explains the full nature and severity of their problem, you should expect little else. Other patients drop out because they resent the impersonal treatment during the early stages of care when they complied with your every request through gritted teeth. Still others resent the price placed on what appears to be a very simple procedure, at a time when they're feeling fine.

Lack of referrals: While many patients report exasperation at trying to motivate friends or family members, all too many patients don't even try. Some have felt used, treated like a number, or don't wish others to know they've consulted a charismatic cult figure. Still others don't refer because they resent being put on the spot to reveal the name of "someone else who needs chiropractic care." The best restaurants, the best hair stylists, and the best doctors don't have to ask for referrals. Consistently exceed patient expectations and the referral process will take care of itself.

Narrow understanding: When you honor your patients you naturally want to educate them. Not only does patient education generate more respect for the doctor, patient education empowers patients. Information is power. Volunteering information tells patients that you think they're important because responsible people want to know "why?"

Ultimately, if you're going to honor the patient you must communicate with the patient in the most powerful ways possible. All too often we depend upon some of the least effective and superficial dimensions:

Kinesthetically: This is the easiest level on which to communicate with patients and the one to which patients are most apt to succumb. "How do you feel?" you ask brightly as you enter the adjusting room. Doctors who put an overemphasis on symptoms or the relief of symptoms, convince patients that how they feel is the most important thing they're interested in. These practices are basically pain clinics that lack the satisfaction that comes from long term relationships with their "clients."

Intellectually: Here, the analytical approach reigns, working under the assumption that if patients just knew enough, they'd make the right decisions about their health (long term wellness care). While patient education is important, it takes more. Communicating at this level, while on a higher plane than the "feeling" approach, still lacks the depth that long term relationships are made of.

Financially: In the past, all too many doctors have looked to what an insurance policy will pay to determine the treatment program. Offices too interested in what an attorney thinks can be extracted from an insurance carrier or are quick to push the limits of what a job related injury can generate, have lowered themselves to "X-raying the patients wallet." It gives chiropractic a black eye.

More effective communication centers around more powerful issues. Like a double-edged sword, these issues are often avoided. Fearing that patients would reject them or find these topics too personal, they are overlooked. Too bad. Because spoken or unspoken, the deepest and most secure doctor/patient relationships include or address these topics in some way.

Values: Look at the person you married or the friends that you've had for years and you'll find shared values. You may not agree on everything, but what makes long term relationships last is shared values. Of course, if you don't know what your values are, it's difficult to share them with others. And you needn't be oppressive about it. The key is to reveal enough so patients know where you stand on various issues of the day. How do you feel about government, politics, education, the media, and related issues. Abandon the myth that you have to be all things to all people. Take a stand.

Spirituality: Sprinkle your conversation with clues about your spiritual beliefs. Not that you're going to change someone's religion in the adjusting room, but volunteer your perspective when opportunities present themselves. It might be as simple as placing a Bible in the reception room, wearing a piece of jewelry, or revealing some other "clue." Create opportunities for patients to start a conversation about spiritual matters.

Not all patients want a deep relationship with their doctors, so be careful. Like in any relationship, a patient can be "blown away" by moving too quickly or revealing too much. The point is to become more vulnerable and open with patients who seem hungry for a more meaningful relationship. That doesn't mean you become pals. It means stepping down from your pedestal or soapbox long enough to be a real person. Doing so is the mark of the personal and professional self-confidence that most patients find attractive. ∎

REVEALING ONE'S CHIROPRACTIC IDENTITY

It's a well-accepted axiom that the best patients are those who are referred to your office. When an existing patient vouches for you and sends friends or family members to your office they, are usually more predisposed to your procedures and recommendations. Based on the trust they have for their friend's judgment, the new patient is usually less apprehensive and more willing to participate in your office routines. Because patients who are referred to your office generally respect you and are more enjoyable to treat, increasing the number of new patient referrals is a major, albeit rarely spoken aloud goal of most offices. Yet, by virtue of the fact that referrals require current or previously active patients to reveal their chiropractic experience (peer pressure), defend their decision (overcome the myths about chiropractors), and convince others (patient education), referrals are a rare commodity in many offices.

Unlike paid for advertising, word-of-mouth advertising, because it is apparently out of the control and influence of the practitioner, is the most powerful and trusted form of marketing. However, it is much more within your control than you think, especially if you see this process from the patient's perspective! Here are some observations and specific action steps you might take to increase the likelihood that your patients will be ready, willing, and able to tell others about your office.

Peer pressure: Since you live so deeply within the chiropractic subculture it is often difficult to see the unwillingness many patients have to reveal their chiropractic identity to others. Many of today's image-conscious patients are reluctant to admit to their friends or work associates that they have consulted an alternative-not-approved-cult healer. Over the years this has generated millions of chiropractic patients who received results but haven't told anyone about their experience. This "chiropractic underground" has created an artificial barrier to the acceptance and growth of chiropractic. It is one of the reasons why it takes more than being a great clinician to have a great practice.

Patients who worry about wearing the right brand name jeans, driving the right imported automobile, and wondering what the neighbors think, may be reluctant to tell others about their brush with a non-mainstream health care practitioner. Perhaps those of lower socio-economic status are not so reticent to admit to others they've been to a "doctor" who advertises in the yellow pages, chases people down the mall with a plastic spine, or apparently has to advertise on television with personal injury lawyers and waterbed discounters.

Action steps. Create an office environment that reflects better taste than brown carpet with 1972 Motel Six vinyl chairs. Employ office procedures that are respectful of the patient. Locate your office in an area that affirms your professional mainstream perspective. Don't confront your patients to reveal names of their friends that "need chiropractic care." Avoid badgering patients to continue coming in after their perceived needs have been met. In other words, make sure you treat patients with at least the same dignity they would get when consulting any other licensed professional. Make sure that your patients can tell others that you're "not like all those other chiropractors."

Overcome chiropractic myths: Because virtually all North Americans have been influenced by the media, the A.M.A., low budget television commercials, insurance claims adjusters, bent pens, no out of pocket expense advertising, and the other collective misjudgments of this profession of Lone Rangers, misconceptions about chiropractic abound. The perceived unscientific nature of chiropractic, the lack of education, the possibility of stroke or paralysis, and the notion that once you start chiropractic care you'll get addicted to adjustments and need them forever, are powerful and lingering myths that haunt many in our culture. Even some of your best patients harbor these notions. Because many patients are ill-equipped to explain away this bigotry or overcome the conventional wisdom about chiropractic, it's easier not to try. That's one reason many don't expose their involvement with chiropractic to others.

Remember, these notions often exist even in the face of a miracle cure or extraordinary clinical results. Even patients who are the most loyal and compliant can harbor these misconceptions about chiropractic. Certainly patients must experience results from your care to endorse you to others, but if they can't overcome the myths others have, they won't be as successful in referring others.

Action steps. Start by asking new patients what they've heard about chiropractic. Try to determine where they stand and what their "pre-existing condition" is regarding chiropractic. Make a list of the most common myths and misconceptions about the profession and create a patient handout or have a staff member clear up these issues during the early part of care. No need to take a defensive posture, merely present them with "information that our new patients want to know." After several visits ask patients what their greatest fear or misconception about chiropractic was when they called for that first appointment. Make sure on subsequent visits that you supply information that will equip them to put this issue to rest if it is raised by a friend or family member.

Convince others: Sadly, even after getting great results, many chiropractic patients are powerless to describe the purpose, procedures, and practice of chiropractic. It is inexcusable that patients who have been in the office for as many visits as the most generous insurance policy accommodates still can't describe what a subluxation is, which of their legs is long or short, what an adjustment is, what the sound is, and why chiropractic works. Since these chiropractic basics are unlikely to get media coverage, it's up to each doctor to provide adequate patient education if he or she expects referrals.

Most everyone can explain what happens at the dentist; even what an appendectomy is. Yet many of your best patients are without the language or understanding to explain what happens on a typical visit in your office! For too many patients, their care is something that happens to them and apparently works. This superficial experience prevents many from feeling confident enough to explain chiropractic to others contemplating care. It makes it difficult to answer the inevitable questions and make a convincing case to those suffering from low back pain at work or headaches at home. Patient education empowers patients to be better chiropractic advocates.

Action steps. Obviously patient education must be a consistent process. Systematize your efforts. Pick a new topic each day and relate the patient's problem to this subject. Make it relevant. Include these types of brief "factoids" in your newsletters. Put an educational message on your sign in sheet. Give patient lectures. Use videos. Ask patients how they describe different aspects of chiropractic and their care to others. Don't become a bore, but accept your responsibility to be a good steward of your knowledge and clinical experience. If they don't learn it from you, they won't learn it—thwarting the referral process.

Finally, there's one other important factor affecting the referral process. Few talk about it because it is the most fundamentally difficult to change. It's you. Are you worthy of your patients' trust? Are you someone your patients are willing to endorse? Do you have a personality? Are you communicative? Are you a superb listener? Are you trustworthy?

Would you rather be flown by a pilot that explains why you're parked motionless on the tarmac or by one who is silent? Would you rather be served by a waitress that volunteers what's good on the menu today or by one who merely takes your order? Would you rather work for a boss that involves you in decisions that affect your job responsibilities or by one who ignores you? Would you rather be treated by a doctor who is upbeat and optimistic or by one who seems preoccupied and distant? Both pilots, waitpersons, bosses, and doctors may be of equal skill and experience, yet the passenger, customer, employee, and patient perceives the more external and communicative professional as being better. It may not be fair, and this subtle aspect of the doctor/patient relationship may be ignored in chiropractic colleges, yet it may be one of the most important aspects of a successful chiropractic career. It creates delighted patients and the effortless stimulation of the referral process. ■

EXTRAORDINARY PATIENT CARE

For many doctors, the reasons why many patients don't refer remains a continual mystery. "I tell my friends, but they won't come in," observes an apparently satisfied patient. This is a common response by those who *are* telling others. Unfortunately, all too many patients, even satisfied patients, just don't tell anyone about their experience. This puts the office on a stressful treadmill, constantly searching for new patients through advertising, aggressive telemarketing efforts, or image-endangering flea market spinal screenings. Treating the symptoms of a lack of new patients in this way, overlooks the internal office shortcomings that may be sabotaging the referral process. Avoiding the truth is an all too common affliction of many doctors–especially those who most want to maximize their practice potential.

There is this misguided notion that if you can avoid office problems, ignore occasionally mentioned patient disappointments, or look past the symptoms of poor patient rapport, they will somehow go away. If the patient doesn't "get it," the patient is blamed. If patients discontinue care before optimum healing has been reached, we seldom look in the mirror for the cause. Somehow the patient, the staff, the insurance company, or some other defect is targeted for blame.

Sometimes we're just too busy. Or we aren't hungry enough. Or we're oblivious to the fact that we haven't "connected." Still other times we aren't sensitive enough to detect the early signs of impending dropout in time to prevent it. Often the things we know will work are only deployed when sufficiently low patient volume necessitates it. Most of the time we would rather try some new gadget or thingamajig that won't require the energy demanded of things we *know* will work.

There are no shortcuts. You have probably already implemented all the "easy" ways to grow your practice.

Few will disagree that a regular public speaking outreach program will almost automatically grow your practice. But that requires too much energy or confronting a fear. "What I'm looking for, is something I can buy for less than $500, plug into the wall, and get new patients without effort," smiles a doctor voicing the unadmitted fantasy of all too many struggling offices. Too bad.

As chiropractic care enters a market economy, influenced by a revolutionary concept called "supply and demand," doctors that survive the shedding of low insurance deductibles will notice that they must become increasingly creative in their communication, tableside manners, financial policy, accessibility, and office environment. No longer will a 1200 square foot "bowling alley" shaped office in a "shopette" with a high traffic count guarantee success. It is going to take more energy and more attention to detail to create and maintain an office that is effective, fun, and continually interesting for patients (and you) to want to return to again and again and again.

If your notion of practice is spending endless hours of orgasmic delight, adjusting one grateful patient after another without dealing with nonclinical issues, dream on. And while it's sad that most chiropractic colleges and technique seminars have made new graduates focus on the adjustment, the doctor's adjusting prowess is rarely mentioned in patient focus groups. As long as the doctor doesn't hurt the patient and patients get the symptomatic results they want, most are satisfied. Yet, mere satisfaction is not how you grow a practice from the inside out through the referral process! Growth requires patients who leave the practice on every visit delighted, enthusiastic, proud, and ecstatic–characteristics that usually take more to elicit than a smartly administered lumbar roll between the weather and sports scores!

As I tour more and more offices, I've seen some things that patients tend to talk about at focus groups. These procedures and personal touches contribute to patients adopting a long-term chiropractic lifestyle. They are small things that might not have been worth it at a time when countless $100 deductibles stood ready at your door, complying with your offer for free services. Today, in a world of "niche" marketing, Faith Popcorn's "egonomics," and interest in the burgeoning wellness segment of health care, new approaches are necessary.

What would patients deem extraordinary? Depends who your patients are and what their expectations are. Blue collar workers, still in their work uniforms, have a different idea of what would be extraordinary than perhaps the mother with two energetic toddlers. Regardless of who your patients are (or who you'd like them to be), here are some ideas to consider:

Call after first adjustment: An old idea that works just as well as it did 20 years ago. Most doctors overlook this important rapport-building opportunity because they aren't prepared to handle any potential negative feedback. Practice how you'd answer the three potential answers, "I feel better," "I feel no change," and "I feel worse." Then, astound your new patients with a phone call that demonstrates you really care.

Unusual magazine selection: Office reading material is frequently mentioned in patient focus groups. Offer reading material that is upbeat, optimistic, and highly-visual. Locate interesting, creative magazines that patients don't see waiting in line at the grocery store check-out counter.

Interesting music: Avoid using the radio to set the mood of your office. If all you play is Top 40, golden oldies, or elevator music, you're missing an important opportunity to actively set the "tone" of your office. Get a CD player and locate instrumental music that is soothing and can't be heard in the patient's car driving to your office.

Anticipating patient needs or fears: Think back to a fantastic dinner in a great restaurant. A common feature of extraordinary service, where ever it is encountered, is when the customer's needs are anticipated. Volunteer information about the sound the drop pieces are making. Volunteer how you reduce X-ray exposure and all the other things you do to make a patient's care safe. If you wait for them to ask the question, regardless of your answer, it won't be extraordinary. Anticipation is the key.

Patient education: It's overlooked, but educating your patients, whether it's through lectures, videos, or systematic adjusting room banter, is extraordinary. It is special only because their medical doctor rarely takes the time. Most of today's patients want to participate more directly in their care program and have questions. Providing information shows you really care.

Offering emergency phone number: While this is sometimes relegated to monotone pronouncements on the office telephone answering machine, being more aggressive in revealing your willingness to help patients during hours the clinic is closed, communicates a strong message of service. Don't worry, few will take you up on your offer. Those who do will be grateful and often enthusiastic in ways quite beneficial to the office.

Special hours: Do you have hours like every other doctor? Extraordinary offices design their practice hours around the accessibility needs of their patients, balanced with the need to have a life, too. Maybe stay open late or start early one day a week. Danger: Changing your office hours too frequently becomes a sore spot with patients. There are certain issues like hours and adjusting technique that patients want predictability.

Remembering patient volunteered information: If you want to astound patients, keep good records of the little comments they make or things that are happening in their lives that they mention. Make a note on the travel card. If the staff hears something, make sure they mention it to you, too. This is a powerful demonstration of your listening skills and your interest in caring for the total person, not just their spine.

Be a community referral resource: As a doctor, working with a variety of people, you have the opportunity to be a clearing house of information about other businesses and service providers. Obviously recommend painters, contractors, printers, and other tradespeople who are your patients. You might avoid putting up everyone's business card on the bulletin board, but there are other ways you can let it be known that you "have friends" that might be able to help them. (Does this idea make you uncomfortable? Remember, you're asking your current patients to do the same thing with their friends!)

Reception room telephone: Again, it's a small thing, but if patients are always asking to use a phone, consider installing one in the reception area. You can have long distance calls blocked so all it costs is a nominal line access charge each month. No one said providing extraordinary service was going to be free.

Scenting the headrest paper: If you want patients to look forward to their care and have some fun in the process, consider scenting your headrest paper. Vanilla, chocolate, and other more exotic flavors are available in small vials at stores that specialize in fragrances. (Avoid stressful "mint" type aromas as well as coconut—patients may think they are smelling some other patient's suntan lotion.)

Family fee arrangements: With good patient education you create a demand for delighted patients to bring their families in for care. However, even as extraordinary as your care may be, if a family has too much difficulty fitting chiropractic into their budget, they won't. Create a variety of financial alternatives, a menu of ways whole families can afford care in your office. Special fees for kids?

Interesting toy box: Speaking of kids, how about an extraordinary experience for children? A great toy box, not filled with the broken hand-me-down parts your kids don't want anymore, but some great toys, can serve to attract families to your office. Appealing to kids seems to work for McDonald's.

Raising patients' self esteem: If you could improve each patient's perception of him or herself by simply being in your presence, you wouldn't have a compliance problem! "Oh, you look so good in blue." "I just love seeing your name on the appointment book because I know I'm going to see your smiling face." The list is endless. As long as you mean it, it can help your patients look forward to showing up for their dose of encouragement and appreciation.

As you delight and exceed your patients' expectations by employing some of these ideas, realize that after time, things that used to exceed their expectations, now have become expected! So besides the demands of constantly meeting their expectations, you must rise to the challenge of setting new, ever higher standards. If you thought you could ever rest on your laurels or coast, you should have gone to work for the post office. ■

THE MUSIC OF HEALING

An often overlooked aspect of creating the optimum office environment is the music that emanates from the speakers in the ceiling. Music is very personal. It is not unusual to find two or three different radios throughout a chiropractic office, responding to the particular tastes of the listeners. Everything from golden oldies to country western twang to babbling talk radio hosts can be heard by patients, depending upon whether they're waiting, getting adjusted, or resolving financial matters. Office music is a topic frequently mentioned by patients in focus groups. Music is an opportunity to take an active role in shaping the "tone" of your office.

Research suggests that music can play a profound role in the healing process and overall good health. Music can help avoid depression, improve immune system response, raise self-esteem, and affect other aspects important in the recovery of one's health. On a personal level, music can be very affirming. Many of us have certain kinds of music we like to listen to when we're relaxing, when we're driving our car, or when we want to create a romantic evening. As teenagers, we used music to rebel against our parents. Today we use music (and how loud we play it) to provide a backdrop for our lifestyles, reflecting our mood.

Music can add energy to a slow morning and music can play a role in mellowing out a hectic evening rush hour. Depending upon some 26 year-old who is living at home in his parents basement, who programs the local easy listening radio station, isn't good enough. Music is one way to demonstrate to patients that you're on top of the details. Plus, the right music can make each day a lot more enjoyable for the doctor and staff.

Many of us associate major events in our lives with the music we were listening to at the time. Because of circumstances, I happen to associate negative feelings with *Moon River* by Andy Williams and just about anything by the Carpenters. I have especially fond memories attached to James Taylor's *Fire and Rain* and *Momma Told Me Not To Come* by a group whose name escapes me today. Most of us have these negative and positive associations with specific songs or types of music and will change stations or turn up the volume when we hear them. Your patients have these types of associations, too. If you play commercial Top 40 radio or music from the 60s and 70s in your office (complete with spots for Preparation H and Nuprin), you run the risk of resurrecting memories in your patients that may be counterproductive to your overall intent. Plus, relying on standard issue music that patients can get by turning on their own car radio on their way to your office doesn't make their office experience exceptional or extraordinary. Music, when thoughtfully chosen, can be used to enhance the office experience of your patients.

One of the greatest myths circulating in chiropractic is that when creating your office you should be careful not to offend anyone. Perhaps this is why most chiropractic offices resemble medical doctor offices. The result is an office that is bland and lacks personality. Patients feel little connection with the office—and neither does the staff. To attract patients like yourself, take opportunities to reveal things you like. Like the music in your office. Unless your tastes are limited to Tasmanian ritual drum music, you'll probably find ample numbers of people who like what you like. Here are some considerations when selecting music for your office:

No lyrics: Besides avoiding memory-filled music from the past or instrumental versions of well known tunes that we're inclined to hum along with, consider new music. Look for music that your patients may have never heard before. Remember, the objective of music is to be in the background, setting the tone of the office. Use music with a gentle rhythm and tones that project harmony and unity. While for some the term "New Age" may have negative connotations, the interesting, yet soothing music you're looking for can often be found in this section of the music store.

Use CDs: The compact disc has made buying music a lifetime investment. No scratches. Perfect reproduction. Small. And easy to use. Your one-time purchase will last for the rest of your life. I prefer CDs over cassette tapes because of a feature found on many CD players that makes it the perfect vehicle for your office: shuffle play. Shuffle play is a term used by Sony, but other manufacturers offer players with the same ability to randomly play various cuts on as many as six different discs. Unlike audio cassettes or vinyl albums which we "learn" to anticipate the next tune, employing this randomizing option helps keep each disc fresh and new. You may want to get a set of discs that has a more energetic tone for the mornings and a different set that is more restful for the afternoon and evening hours.

Monaural: This is a little detail that is often overlooked by the do-it-yourselfer who installs his or her own office music system. Be sure to combine both left and right signals of the output of your amplifier so that every speaker has both channels of information! Otherwise, patients may hear only half of the music.

Volume control: This is a feature that many doctors wish they had installed after living with their sound system for a while. If you're going to play music in all areas of your office, you may want the ability to control the volume in treatment areas differently than in the more "public" areas of your office such as the reception area and hallways. If adding individual volume controls isn't possible at this stage, there are speaker manufacturers that have volume controls mounted on the grill for this purpose.

When I address the concepts of office music in seminars, I invariably get questions about those "chiropractic commercials" that can be interspersed with the music. The idea here is to subtly brainwash patients through the "big brother" speakers in the ceiling. Apparently this rationale is based on the notion that we've given up on direct approaches for educating patients. When using this method, the public address system in the office has changed from shaping the tone of the office on an unconscious level, to manipulating a patient by directing their attention without their consent. This is the same frustration patients feel when they are forced to wait in reception areas that only have chiropractic-oriented reading material. These chiropractic commercials are probably more appropriate for patients to listen to while they are holding on the telephone. The only problem is, superior patient service would suggest patients shouldn't be asked to hold long enough to get a meaningfully complete message.

Interestingly, the most effective types of music for the office aren't obvious. Music contributes to a feeling about the office, the doctor, the procedures, and atmosphere by being in the background. When it becomes the central issue of complaints or comments by patients, or when the doctor and staff place too much emphasis on it, something's not right. Keep working at it.

There are several legal issues at work here you should be aware of. Strict enforcement of copyright laws would suggest that playing music in your office is a "performance." Currently, the two largest firms that collect royalties for composers and performers, ASCAP and BMI, are turning their heads when it comes to using prerecorded music in a professional setting. Restaurants, shopping centers, and other very public areas that use music have already had to toe the line, producing many "canned music" suppliers that own performance rights and lease the music to businesses via a monthly fee. These services distribute the music on special long playing 8-track tapes or by satellite. However, my conversations with ASCAP suggest little interest in clamping down on professional office use of the radio, audio cassette, or CD performances.

I've been auditioning some music that might serve as a head start for finding music appropriate for your healing environment. Here are a few of my favorites: *Sedona Suite* by Tom Barabas, *Reflections of Passion*, by Yanni, *Feather Light* by Hilary Stagg, *The Light of the Spirit* by Kitaro, *Shepherd Moons* and *Watermark* by Enya. ■

MAKING
CHIROPRACTIC VALUABLE

You're doing your shopping at the supermarket after forgetting your shopping list. You do the best you can, pausing here and there, attempting to remember what you need and don't need. Between the paper towels and napkins you pause in front of the bathroom tissue. Was bathroom tissue on the list? Four rolls of two-ply is priced at $1.09. After a slight hesitation you decide bathroom tissue wasn't on the list and you finish filling up your shopping cart.

Upon reaching home you're dismayed to learn that bathroom tissue *was* on your list. In moments you're back in your car. However, this time you're not going to the mega-mart with built-in bakery, fish market, and video rentals. This time you're headed to the open-24-hours-a-day convenience mart!

Pulling into the lot, you grab a parking spot just 20 feet from the door. Thankfully, you take the few steps to the rear of the store and reach for the same four roll, 2-ply package of your favorite national brand bathroom tissue you saw at the supermarket. The price? Fifty cents more at $1.59. Without hesitation, you take the object of your desire to the checkout counter and give the cashier $2.00, get your change, and seconds later you're back in the car heading home. The extra 50 cents was paid for the added value of the convenience that was bundled with the bathroom tissue. It was paid after making the decision that avoiding the two-mile parking lot hike, and the mother standing in line having a power struggle with her four-year old, was worth the extra half buck. It was the same bathroom tissue, yet its access and convenience made it "worth" more. In other words, the convenience was a "value" or quality that was added to the price.

In a chiropractic setting it's tempting to lower fees and disregard the option of adding more value instead. In fact, the whole issue of compliance and the dismay many doctors felt in the 1980's, when they encountered a cash patient, is directly related to being able to create or add value to a patient's chiropractic experience. Just about everyone can afford chiropractic care, it's just that they value their annual ski weekends to Colorado or driving a late model car even more.

The path of least resistance is to lower the fees, or make special "deals" that clutter the books and make it difficult for staff members to collect fees and administer the financial policy. Worse, when patients talk, as they often do, and find out Mrs. Smith is only paying $XX per adjustment, tempers can flare and doubts about the doctor's integrity arise.

Lowering fees is almost always just an expedient way to treat a *symptom*. The *cause* is a lack of value communicated by the doctor, or of not adding enough value to the experience of receiving their care. This seems especially difficult for doctors to do when patients are relieved of their pain, or their most obvious symptoms have cleared up.

Perhaps it is because of this, that there is still a sizable contingent of chiropractic doctors who don't "believe" in non-symptomatic care. They observe that without obvious symptoms, there is no need for chiropractic adjustments. Plus, insurance companies don't pay for that sort of care anyway. Why bother?

First, these are the same doctors who for the last ten years, have gotten adjusted at least once a month themselves, sometimes more often. Second, only treating patients with obvious symptoms (and insurance policies) is a stressful and limited way to serve the community, ignoring children and preventive care. Third, avoiding the self-esteem-wrenching confrontation required of a doctor to place a value on what his or her (nonsymptomatic) care is worth, in favor of personal injury, workers compensation, and major medical patients, transfers an inordinate and inappropriate amount of control to third parties.

The issue here is value. When patients, even cash paying patients, are receiving the symptomatic relief they desire during the earliest stages of their care, there are usually few problems with patient compliance. Patients get value for their financial exchange. It usually isn't until later, when they're feeling better, that the lack of perceived value starts to emerge. The seeds for this patient rebellion are often sown on the first visit and reinforced throughout their experience in the office.

It often starts by the doctor or office staff communicating in many subtle ways, how delighted they are to have the patient. With new patient volume down in so many offices these days, this is more of a problem than it used to be. When you forget that patients need you a whole lot more than you need the patient, you fall into a leadership trap that comes back to bite you later. Allowing patients to dictate what you will and won't do (take X-rays, adjust on the first visit, etc.) further erodes their confidence and endangers the leadership role you'll need even more, later.

Another subtle way some doctors sabotage their ability to effectively communicate value to their patients later, when they're feeling better, is to focus their chiropractic explanations around the concept of misalignments instead of spinal malfunction. (Ironically, these are the same doctors unwilling to document the effectiveness of their regimen with post-X-rays!) That's a dangerous double standard. Worse, doctors can get into trouble when symptomatic patients present themselves with proper spinal curves and apparent subluxation-free static views. It is easier to explain the necessity of continued non-symptomatic visits, if a dynamic model of spinal function is used instead. Here, functional X-rays, and the related non-symptomatic muscle and soft tissue involvement, make a stronger case to patients.

Yet, the most overlooked issue that lowers the value patients will place on their chiropractic care, is the health of their chiropractor. If you're overweight, still smoking, or sanction these and other poor health habits in your staff, you have a credibility problem. The "do-as-I-say, not-as-I-do" school of patient management isn't as effective as it once was. Setting a good example is important. "If the doctor doesn't value his health, why should I?" reasons a patient. "If she isn't going to follow her own advice, why should I?" justifies another patient. "Obviously chiropractic doesn't work," surmises another.

Adding value to the patient's chiropractic experience takes more than simply avoiding certain mistakes. It takes a conscious effort and a willingness to persevere, even in light of outright patient rejection or the lack of instant gratification. All of the following suggestions require extra time, energy, or worse yet, change. They are often common denominators of those doctors able to "collect the extra 50 cents" during a recession, or see a full patient load during a winter snowstorm. Do you have the discipline and courage that's needed?

Relentless patient education: These doctors never stop! Videos and brochures? Of course. Lectures, orientations, and chiropractic topic-of-the-day, further round out their efforts. Without being a bore, they're always talking chiropractic with their patients. These doctors recognize that patients will not go to chiropractic college or be able to trust the media to expand their patients' understanding of chiropractic principles. They take their responsibility seriously.

Interesting environment: The doctor must show respect for chiropractic and themselves before patients will. Adding value to the patients' perceptions starts with their first impressions upon entering the office, and continues through a series of many visits. Unlike a sterile, unchanging medical doctor-type office, creating an interesting environment is crucial in demonstrating value for patients. If the doctor doesn't think chiropractic is important, exhibited in tangible terms by the office he or she practices in, patients won't think chiropractic is valuable either. That doesn't mean you create a showplace and leave it alone! It means constantly romancing the bulletin boards, updating the magazine rack with new and interesting titles, introducing new toys, and giving the entire office a continual facelift. If you want patients to return again and again, it must be interesting, stimulating, and have an "up" tone.

A passionate doctor: Patient education, office environment, and other aspects described here, share this one element in common; the doctor is excited and committed to chiropractic. It's hard to add value to a patient's experience, if the doctor projects a black cloud from burnout or financial pressures. Patients can tell when the doctor isn't having "fun" and that the practice is work. They can "smell" the doctor's stress and the constant fixation of getting more new patients. Patients (or staff members) are rarely more excited about chiropractic than the doctor.

Attach to patient's key value: One important and frequently overlooked way to increase a patient's value of chiropractic, is to help them more directly associate their care with something they *do* value. Are you finding out what they hope to do better or enjoy more upon regaining their health through chiropractic? It shouldn't take too much creativity to associate the need for continued adjustments (even non-symptomatic adjustments) with being able to sleep through the night, improve their golf game, or be able to lift up their grandchildren. Refresh the patient's memory that this is why they're continuing to show up in your office on subsequent office visits. Before you begin their care, ask patients why they want improved health.

Crediting the patient: While your ego craves the affirmation that producing chiropractic results so frequently offers, turn it around. Help patients realize you are merely a facilitator for their body's own inborn healing potential. Adding value this way is not only more honest, it shows that you're in partnership with their bodies. This anchors their chiropractic experience at a deeper, more fundamental level than that of a self-indulgent luxury or a "can-I-afford-it?" extravagance.

Short waiting time: It's not just the financial cost of care that can discourage continued care, it is also the cost in terms of the time. Time is the new luxury commodity. If your office hours are inconvenient for the plant workers down the highway, it can interfere with their visit schedule. If parking is a problem, your lack of parking may be affecting patient compliance. Like the convenience store around the corner, removing barriers to the access of your office is essential in the drive-up-window-microwave-world we live in today.

Let's face it. There are some patients, like horses led to water who won't drink, that have little inclination to continue their care into a preventive or wellness mode. So while you aren't likely to connect with everyone, you owe patients at least some explanation of the value of continued care.

The point is, to add value to a patient's chiropractic experience before taking the easy route of lowering your fees. Ironically, the most common result reported by those who lower their fees, is a drop in their income! Lowering your fees will not automatically increase your patient volume. Without adding some form of value, you could *give* your care away and still have an empty appointment book.

The problem in most offices isn't the fee structure. It's an issue of *value*. After all, how many of those convenience stores with the expensive bathroom tissue have you seen go out of business? ∎

CONVERTING THE
PI PRACTICE

As more and more doctors read the hand writing on the wall, they are coming to the conclusion that the "golden goose" of plentiful worker's comp and personal injury cases is about to migrate south. Those that "got while the getting was good" made a very nice living. Lots of patients. The right to advertise. Abundant insurance money. Helpful lawyers. And a chance to repeatedly prove to oneself with a constant stream of symptomatic patients that chiropractic works.

Today an increasing number of legislatures are finding that the disorganization and infighting often characterizing the chiropractic profession are easy targets dealing with burdensome worker's compensation problems. Capping chiropractic care at twelve visits, requiring a medical referral for continued treatment, the right of the employer to select the treating doctor, and other similar tactics that victimize the patient, have significantly modified the practice environment.

Even the lucrative area of personal injury is finding lawsuit amounts limited by some state laws. Lawyers who were "friends of chiropractic" are finding their case load dropping. Have you reviewed the lawyer section in the telephone yellow page directory recently? It looks a lot like the chiropractic section did in the late 1980s. With more and more lawyers chasing fewer and fewer "good" cases, their shark-like instincts are turning to a source of income: doctor malpractice. These days you don't know whether your next new patient is an insurance company plant, a television investigative reporter, or someone teamed up with a hungry lawyer attempting to catch you making a mistake! "You mean the doctor didn't _____? I think we've got a malpractice case on our hands."

While certain aspects of the good old days remain, many doctors are hedging their bets and are beginning to convert their practices over to more of a cash-paying family practice. And while it seems like a transition from one to the other should be a simple matter, many doctors are finding it difficult, especially in light of the financial dynamics of the times. If you're contemplating making this type of change in your practice, here are some things to ponder:

Headspace: Clearly, patients who show up in your office due to a work related injury have an entirely different motive than patients who are self-directed and show up in your office and pay cash. The first element in a successful transition is adopting a new perspective about your patients. No longer can they be seen as a $1500 or higher case fee, they must be nurtured in the style of the family doctor. Those who possess the fatherly Rockwellesque qualities of being a good listener with seemingly endless amounts of time will have an easier go.

Frequently patients who pay out of their own pockets have different expectations than those who are in the office for pain relief so they can keep their job. Being able to identify and match these expectations is critical to establishing rapport and the long term relationship that is often possible. First and foremost it starts with the doctor's attitude and vision for the future.

Patient education: In the workers comp/PI environment, patient education is usually no more ambitious than stressing the importance of keeping the appropriate visit schedule. When their care is being paid for by "someone else" this modest amount of patient education is usually enough to get the patient through the initial stages of care and symptomatic relief. Never mind that damaged soft tissues haven't been rehabilitated, leaving the patient susceptible to a relapse (that they'll blame you for)!

When patients have to reach into their back pocket on every visit, they demand better answers. Don't be misled by the patients who aren't brave enough to reveal their lack of knowledge by boldly asking questions. If you want more families in your office you must consistently *volunteer* information and *anticipate* their concerns.

Fee structure: Which brings up the most difficult aspect of creating a family practice: fees. Cash paying patients, especially families, seem unwilling to pay what you have been able to extract from the deep pockets of an insurance company. The prospect of having to see more patients to make up for the loss of income is often too challenging for doctors in their sixth or tenth year of practice who were hoping to sit back and "coast" at this stage in their career. This is where many doctors turn back and decide fighting over the dwindling amount of insurance money will be just fine.

Don't get discouraged! If you're tired of fighting insurance companies and writing apparently ignored narrative reports and waiting months, sometimes years for payment, cash-paying families sound pretty attractive. Remember, you don't have to go cold turkey. Spend the next year or so in a slow transition.

Pediatrics: Funny how a screaming but helpless little child can strike fear in the hearts of the biggest, strongest chiropractor. If you want to move out of symptom-treating insurance cases into a cash-paying family practice you've got to become proficient with adjusting children. Many post-graduate and seminar programs exist to help the doctor make this a reality. There are solutions to virtually every fear you have about adjusting newborns, infants, or children of all ages. Do it!

Office environment: I've seen family practices with PI and worker's comp cases, but I haven't seen too many PI and worker's comp practices with lots of families. What seems to happen in a lot of the insurance-mill type practices is that the office environment takes on a utilitarian, uninspired appearance. Instead of regularly reinvesting in the office furnishings, colors, and accessories, the office is consumed with patient volume. Aesthetics, professional image, and patient comfort take a back seat. If you want more families, your office environment may need to be upgraded.

Start with creating a place for children in your office. The number of children in a practice is a good indicator of how healthy the practice is. The more children, the more families, the more fun the doctor and staff are likely to have.

No gimmicks: Advertising seems to work to attract people with spines, but many of the gimmicks and promotional strategies that work to attract insurance-related cases to your practice are less effective when trying to reach families. You are entering a domain that is almost totally controlled by the referral process. That's why patient education, a sparkling personality, and a menu of affordable fee arrangements are so important. You must give patients good reasons for mentioning you to others than the pain relief virtually every patient expects.

Give it time: It takes time to make the transition into a different kind of practice. In many ways it's like starting over. The difference of course is that you already have patients, your school loans aren't nipping at your heels, and you probably have hundreds of inactive patient files sitting on the shelf. But basically you're starting over. How long did it take you to get up to speed when you originally opened your office? Two or three years? Give yourself some time.

A family practice requires that the doctor return to a different era in chiropractic. For those that have become bloated by the easy money of insurance will find the new diet hard to swallow. Those who think they deserve a good living because of their proven healing skills or years of experience may find their reception rooms increasingly empty. Those who are holding out for a national health care plan to save their practice are likely to waste valuable time. The question is, how badly do you want to be a chiropractor? ■

THREE QUESTIONS

Some psychologists believe each of us is motivated by the desire to move toward something (pleasure) or away from something (pain). Knowing what each patient's preferred approach is in the matters of health and personal lifestyle decisions is helpful in formulating the most effective style for communicating with patients. Better communications can improve treatment plan compliance and increase the likelihood that the patient will adopt a chiropractic lifestyle. The degree of success doctors have in motivating patients to embrace the "big idea" of chiropractic is related to their communication skills. Better communicators almost always enjoy more families, children, and the long term relationships of wellness patients in their practices.

In all too many offices there is such an emphasis placed on the patient's physical complaint, and its relief, that the doctor and staff overlook obtaining crucial information that could enhance their ability to "connect" with the patient. While the patient's spine is the primary interest of most doctors, overlooking the patient's preferred communication style invites frustration and misunderstandings. Ignoring the portion of the nervous system enclosed by the skull turns many doctors into mere spine mechanics. Because while some claim only a small percentage of our brain's capacity is used, it is this organ that controls compliance. If the doctor fails to "adjust" this powerful nerve center, he or she will have a limited opportunity to adjust the most vulnerable part of the nervous system below the occiput.

Start by using your new patient admitting form as a means of uncovering a patient's communication style. Do they move toward

71

opportunity or do they attempt to avoid danger? Are they primarily visually, aurally, or kinesthetically oriented? Do they make decisions based on facts or feelings? Knowing the answers could dramatically enhance your communication efforts with each patient.

Using words, when the patient's dominate learning style is by "seeing" invites misunderstanding and a lack of rapport, leading to a lack of confidence in the doctor and premature dismissal. Waxing philosophically about wellness care, optimum function and their fullest potential, when the patient simply wants to avoid pain, is likely to fall on deaf ears. Spouting facts and figures from the latest research projects when the patient makes decisions primarily by how they "feel" about something is a waste of time. The best communicators match the patient's preferred communication style.

Consider adding several multiple choice questions to your admitting paperwork as a way of helping patients reveal their preferred communication modality. Use questions that are seemingly unrelated to their current health complaint so their answers are more likely to reflect their true orientation. Because patients don't expect to find these types of questions on an admitting form, enclose them in a box and explain why you're asking them. Perhaps something like this:

To help us better explain your chiropractic condition and how we may be able to help you, please check the best answer:

1. I remember important things in my life by
   ☐ What I see.
   ☐ What I hear.
   ☐ What I feel.

2. The primary reason I brush my teeth is to
   ☐ Avoid tooth decay and gum disease.
   ☐ Make sure I have healthy teeth and gums.

3. When I make a decision I generally
   ☐ Gather facts and weigh the evidence.
   ☐ Make the right choice instantly.
   ☐ Consult my friends and family.
   ☐ Depend upon how I "feel" about it.

The way patients answer these three simple questions can give you a valuable head start in constructing a more powerful patient report and better adjusting room conversations.

Question #1: The purpose of this question is to find out which "channel" to emphasize in your patient communications. If a patient remembers events with pictures, you'll want to make sure you use images, word pictures, and strong visuals in your communication efforts. If patients remember things by what they hear, you'll want to be sure to offer accurate verbal descriptions of every procedure and conclusion. Perhaps give them an audiotape recording of your report of findings to listen to in the car on the way home. And if patients reveal that they recall a feeling associated with an event, you'll want to make sure you touch the patient, have them hold and touch spinal models, and identify how reduced range of motion feels. Interestingly, most doctors find that patients are visually-oriented, yet the only pictures used in most patient education efforts are static X-rays. No wonder most chiropractic patients think their problem is just a bone out of place!

Question #2: Many patients struggle over this question, yet their answer will provide a valuable insight into how to more effectively present your chiropractic treatment recommendations.

This dental hygiene question is designed to reveal whether the patient prefers to avoid or move away from something (in this case the symptoms of aberrant spinal biomechanics) or towards something (the potential for optimum health and wellness). It is important to match the patients' primary motivator. If they brush their teeth to avoid tooth decay and gum disease, don't expect them to cash in their certificate of deposit at the bank and sign up for your annual Wellness Club! On the other hand, if patients indicate they have a preventive mindset, there's no need to "scare" them into compliance with talk of bone spurs and the expense of a chronic condition, susceptible to relapse. Can this fundamental health attitude be changed? Since our body image is formed at an early age, probably not without huge amounts of time and energy. Speak the language of their current health orientation and, if it's limited, introduce them to the benefits of a preventive outlook as you prove chiropractic "works."

Question #3: The third question reveals a lot about the patient's personality. Are they an Analytical, Driver, Expressive, or Amiable? The first two generally use facts as a basis for making decisions and the second two usually use their feelings. Knowing this important predisposition can better assure that the content of your patient communications has the orientation the patient wants when making decisions about your recommendations.

Make sure your communications to Analyticals and Drivers are complete with research studies, references, statistics, and other facts. Analyticals take longer to make decisions than Drivers, but both are interested in being "right" and will use information packaged as "scientific" in the conclusions they reach. Presenting your report to Expressives and Amiables requires a different tactic. Here, the fact that famous celebrities receive chiropractic care can be effective. So too is the use of metaphors, stories, and emotive "miracle cures."

Knowing the answer to just one of these questions would improve your odds of having meaningful communication with a patient. The real power comes when you combine the information obtained from all three questions. If you discover a patient has a visual orientation, makes decisions based on facts, and tends to move away from problems, you have an important road map you can use to increase rapport and their understanding of chiropractic.

The real test is in using the information you've learned. On the patient's travel card consider printing the words Visual, Aural, Feeling, Towards, Away, Facts. Then, simply circle the appropriate words that reflect the patient's orientation. The circled words will be a constant reminder of how to most effectively communicate with the patient on subsequent visits.

Is this some devious form of brainwashing or patient manipulation? Of course not. It is no different than discovering that a patient prefers a particular adjusting table or appointment time and making that table or time available. Taking the effort to package your patient communications in a way that the patient is predisposed to understand is as polite as hiring a bilingual staff member to assist with certain patients who don't speak English. It's a way of showing respect. Patients will comment that "the doctor knows exactly how I feel" or that "I immediately liked him" or that "I'd been to other chiropractors but no one ever explained it to me before."

Does it take more effort to collect, but more importantly *use* this information? Sure. But you've already done all the easy things to grow your practice! The new frontier, particularly now with increased competition, insurance erosion, and the pressures of managed care, is to keep more patients by turning them into chiropractic clients. And that starts with better patient communications. ■

TUNING IN

I became interested in shortwave radio when I was about ten years old. Each year I would look forward to receiving the Allied Radio Electronics catalog so I could study the full page ad for the Star Roamer shortwave radio. For hours I would stare, mesmerized by the pictures, the specifications (five bands), and imagine the joys of listening to the Voice of America, Radio Moscow, and the BBC World Service. I was intoxicated by this $39.95 radio kit. A lot of money in those days.

One day I hoped to own a Star Roamer and listen in on the world around me. Until then, I studied the pictures and imagined turning the knobs and adjusting my headset.

But there was one knob of the eight on the dial that I couldn't understand. It was labeled "Antenna" and was situated on the left hand side of the radio next to the volume control. I asked my Dad. He didn't know. The antenna knob held my curiosity for over two years until I saved enough of my birthday and lawn mowing money so I could afford to buy a Star Roamer of my own.

When my kit finally arrived, it had to be assembled. Each joint had to be soldered into place and each direction had to be followed precisely.

After I got my kit assembled and rigged a 50 foot wire antenna between the corner of the house and a pole we attached to the fence by the back alley, I finally learned what the antenna knob did. Apparently for optimum reception you need to match the physical length of your antenna with the length of the radio wave frequency you're listening to. But since you can't easily have enough antennas to match every frequency, the antenna knob is used to electronically match the two, improving reception. So after tuning in the station with the big tuning knob, you used the antenna knob for the "fine" tuning. Why didn't they just label the knob "fine tuning?"

I enjoyed years of shortwave radio listening. At the height of the Viet Nam war I wrote a paper for my world history class comparing the reported number of casualties in major battles between Radio Moscow, Radio Havana, and the Armed Forces Radio. All made possible by being able to fine tune my backyard antenna. Understanding patients and "tuning in" to their wants and needs is very similar. It doesn't require a knowledge of Morse Code, but it does require the ability to be sensitive and understand two very important types of patient signals: silence and "Fine."

Most of us are so accustomed to poor service, that our expectations of a dinner out at a new restaurant, working with an architect for the first time, or starting chiropractic care, are fairly low. The poor service we encounter during most of our lives with most service providers has made us so numb, that when things don't live up to our expectations, we often don't even bother telling anyone. "If this is the kind of service they give, why say anything? They're not going to do anything about it anyway," reasons the customer, client, patron, or patient.

Instead of saying something, they just don't come back. And when the subject comes up with friends, they warn them to watch out and avoid the insensitive establishment or practitioner.

Silence is often misconstrued by doctors and other service providers as a meeting of patient expectations. Which is often true. Yet frequently, silence is the refuge taken by those with low self esteem, poor confrontation skills, or those who don't care enough for the doctor's success to mention the shortcomings, misunderstandings, or disappointments. Since no one's complaining about a procedure, a reception room wait, or curt staff member, we figure everything's okay.

"Silence is golden," crowed the Tremolos in their late 1960s hit record, but if you provide any type of service, you know that silence is dangerous. Those with a habit of denying reality needn't bother. Those who bulldoze over patients with esoteric monologues and fill the air with their own agendas need to learn better listening skills. The purpose of this improved sensitivity isn't to become a patient "yes man." The objective is to detect patient satisfaction (or lack of it) and tune your "antenna" to serve as an early warning system to avoid unexplained patient drop out.

One of the most revealing and least threatening ways to take the patient's satisfaction "pulse," is to ask questions. Answering rhetorical, open-ended questions gives patients a platform to express their current physical or psychological health, frustration, or anything else on their minds. Questions like, "So, tell me, what's the best thing that's happened so far today?" "So, if this were your practice, what would you do differently?" "I was wondering, what's the best thing and the worst thing about coming to our office?" "I'm asking all my patients today to rate their experience in our office on a scale of one to one hundred. How would you rate things so far?"

Instead of talking about the weather and sports scores, create informal opportunities for patients to express suggestions, shortcomings, and little pet peeves. You'll probably be delighted by the frequent "everything's just fine" outcomes of these brief interactions and benefit from the occasional identification of easily corrected problems. Getting these rare, but important, less-than-optimum perceptions out into the open can avoid misunderstandings or identify myopic office procedures which hamper both the clinical and non-clinical aspects of your patient relationships.

Moreover, asking these types of questions sets a tone of openness and confidence that patients find attractive. So, even if patients feel reluctant to give you negative feedback while you're cradling their head in your hands, they may be inclined to reveal their impressions to others on the staff. Make sure staff members feel safe in volunteering even the most negative patient comments! Don't shoot the messenger.

Besides patient silence, or not actively offering feedback, tuning into the other dangerous patient signal is equally important. When patients say everything's "fine," it can be a cover-up phrase used to say "I'm-not-willing-to-talk-about-anything-right-now" or at best, it suggests that their minimal expectations are just being met.

At first glance, meeting patient expectations would normally be considered ideal. Yet, referrals and positive word-of-mouth advertising about your practice require that you *exceed* patient expectations. As consumers of services, whether they are chiropractic, car repair, banking, or pizza delivery, we want to be delighted. Yes, we want our problem fixed or our bank account to balance, but exceed our basic expectations by remembering our name, our hobby, our preferred color, or some other small detail about us, and we are impressed. Achieving this level of satisfaction on a non-clinical basis will serve you in ways that a perfectly delivered and technically correct adjustment by itself just can't. In fact, doctors who have mastered this powerful interpersonal aspect of delivering chiropractic care find their practices making a much larger influence in their community than those who graduated with honors, have the perfect office location, or use the latest treatment gizmo.

When patients great you with an "Everything's fine," they just might be telling the truth. But you might want to probe deeper. You may have taken them by surprise, after all, when was the last time a service provider asked you to critique their performance? It's rare. When it does occur, such as a perfunctory, over-the-shoulder jab from a rushed waitperson balancing someone else's meal, telling the truth can be too much of an imposition. Many of us shrug things off, sanctioning less than optimum service, with a smile and a "fine."

Some doctors prefer not knowing what their patients are thinking. The fear that someone will criticize or not like something in which a large emotional investment has been made, forces many into denial. Avoiding feedback opportunities or refusing to create them, isolates you and makes you vulnerable to unexplainable shifts in patient behavior. The unseen blockages to practice growth that plague many offices are quite obvious to patients. Many will tell you, if you'll tune into the right patient frequency by simply asking.

One of the joys of short wave radio listening is tuning into the most distant or weakest signal and requesting a QSL card. After identifying the call letters, frequency, and what was being broadcast at a particular time, listeners write to the shortwave broadcasting station confirming that they have heard the station. A QSL is returned to the listener, usually in the form of a postcard. Besides learning about the world around you, the objective is to collect as many QSL cards as possible. To do so requires the ability to fine tune the signal and eliminate the noise and static. Start "fine" tuning your patients and see patient rapport and compliance improve. ■

WHAT'S NEW?

Seems everyone is always looking for the latest this or the newest that. This constant search for the next gadget or gimmick-of-the-week alarms me. It ignores the fact that the solutions most of us are seeking are already within us. When we look for "new stuff" it is almost always because we are ignoring cause and simply treating a symptom.

Without this yearning, the Western frontier would have remained untamed and the moon untouched. But that's different. When a doctor is awaiting the latest new patient acquisition tool or puts all of his or her hope for the future in a new brochure, video, recall script, or refrigerator magnet, chiropractic is diminished. The doctors I meet who seem to be having the most fun are those who have harnessed the power of their own creativity. Every aspect of their practice reflects their unique personality and philosophy. They are often slow to incorporate the latest gadget.

Mike Vance, who played such an important role in the Disney organization, defines creativity as a "rearranging of the old to create the new." So it's difficult to create if you have little to rearrange. That's why those we brand as "creative" are generally voracious readers, naturally curious and share ideas with those outside their chosen field. Cross-fertilization is important. Besides avoiding the "can't see the forest for the trees" syndrome, many of the challenges facing today's chiropractor have been faced by other professions and industries. Their solutions, while perhaps not automatically transferable, can often stimulate more resourceful thinking in your practice.

In the same way common sense doesn't seem to be all that common these days, many businesses are rediscovering the need to return back to the basics. Increasing numbers of large conglomerates are selling off corporate divisions unrelated to their primary mission. There is an inclination towards simplification. This streamlining, while temporarily negatively affecting the bottom line, restructures the company so it is more focused, more competitive, and ultimately more profitable.

Chiropractic could benefit from this same type of introspection.

What's new in chiropractic? A return to the basics. As insurance crumbles, worker's comp tumbles, managed care becomes more routine, and cost containment becomes the rule, more and more doctors are rediscovering the simplicity and focus that chiropractic enjoyed in the 1960s and early 1970s. Watch that pride and greed don't become twin enemies to your ability to make the adaptation into the future!

Here are the newest and most exciting trends I see for the future:

1. Low overhead: This idea is so new that Greg Stanley of Whitehall Management has been teaching it for over 10 years! Practices that survive and thrive in the 1990s will be those with low overhead. Because you are about to see some incredible price roll-backs in chiropractic, unchaining yourself from a highly-leveraged lifestyle will be critical. No one likes to be the bearer of bad news but watch for the virtual elimination of insurance which could mean as much as a 30% cut in your usual and customary fees. Insurance will still be around. It's just with deductibles as high as your typical case fee, it won't be of much help. Soon, so few patients will have insurance it won't make sense to have the computers, modems, fax machines, and the insurance processing staff to run them. In fact, more and more students emerging from school are already recognizing this. Since they have not been infected by the high, sickness care fees paid by insurance companies, and usually have a modest lifestyle, they have the potential of adapting better than the doctor who has been running a workers comp/PI insurance mill for the last seven years. Cut out the dead wood in your practice.

2. Affordable fees: With the diminishing influence of the insurance industry, doctors will look at their average financial hardship arrangement and devise a relevant fee structure for cash-paying patients. While some will question leaving money on the table when working with the increasingly rare insurance cases, these critics will fail to see the benefits it will afford. Finally the "my-fee-is-my-fee" will start to mean something. It is unlikely you'll need some type of wellness fee structure. The simplicity will make collections easier and close the gap between the ego-deflating difference between services and collections. Thirty-five dollar or higher charges for an adjustment may work for insurance carriers, but in the real world few cash paying patients will pay it. An adjustment may be worth a million bucks, but with an empty reception room other options might be worth exploring.

3. Streamlined procedures: If you've been selling your time (instead of your talent) by conducting long and detailed examinations on every visit, or your adjusting technique is long and drawn out, you may have the biggest adjustment to make. While many justify their detailed diagnostics or elaborate muscle testing because it reveals so much, the return on the patient's investment of time may start exacting too high a price. Spending a lot more time with patients than it takes you to check and adjust your significant other, suggests you're selling your time instead of your talent. Offices that thrive in the future will help patients distinguish the difference. Yes, it requires effective patient communication. However, the best safety net for the uncertain future is a volume practice.

4. Effective patient education: Patients do what they do because they think what they think. If you want more responsible patients now or in the future, effective patient education is essential. You must help patients see chiropractic as a valuable part of their lives, otherwise you become a stressful pain relief clinic. Interestingly, before insurance became such a major influence in chiropractic offices, patient education and the resulting families of patients it created, was an essential ingredient of virtually every office. At a time when there's practically a chiropractor on every corner, it's easy to forget there were doctors who had to build landing strips and hotels by their offices to handle the demand created by their patient education efforts. Help patients "get it." Educated patients are loyal, respectful, and refer others like themselves.

5. Strong philosophy: Ultimately, it boils down to this critical aspect. While the more analytical in the profession try to find research that proves chiropractic works or that nerve interference is real, the rest of the profession quietly goes about its business of facilitating the healing process. Those who are uncomfortable adjusting children miss the real miracles of freeing the life force. Those who mistrust the body or yearn for approval from the allopathic professions are missing the point. The challenge in the 1990s and beyond will be to keep chiropractic distinct and unique in the healing arts. It is and will be the responsibility of every doctor to communicate this unique approach with passion in the most relevant ways possible to those who enter their sphere of influence.

Notice that snappy yellow page ads, thirty-second TV commercials, and reception room marketed water purifiers aren't included in these five essentials. And none of the five "latest trends" in chiropractic depend upon factors outside the four walls of your clinic. In this way you get at the cause of your success or disappointment instead of blaming the weather, traffic patterns, or the number of chiropractors on your block. The future of your practice rests on your ability to read the signs and adapt your style of practice appropriately.

What's new? Committed chiropractors. High impact patient communication. Fee structures that make sense. Appropriate office environments. Serving patients with speed and compassion. Ideas so new, they've been around for a 100 years. ■

INSIDE OUT

The story is told of the Soviet occupation troops showing up in Berlin at the end of World War II who where met by sights that they had never seen before. One soldier, amazed by seeing an electric light bulb for the first time, stood for hours, turning it on, then off again. So impressed with the light, he used his bayonet to cut one down that was hanging from a ceiling. He wanted to take it back home so he could show his family. This is not unlike the popular attitude that many doctors bring with them when they show up at a seminar or convention. "If I can walk away with just one new idea," said a doctor recently, "it'll be worth it." Like the disappointed soldier, many doctors return home and find the videos, posters, scripts, and other "light bulbs" they've harvested from the seminar don't work like they were supposed to.

The doctor isn't to blame. Look around. We've become a "thing" oriented culture. We seem consumed by the newest, latest, and greatest cars, electronics, and other tangible items. While the consumption-oriented, brand name fixation of the past seems to be waning as we start "sacrificing" in the 1990s, all too many of us look to things outside ourselves to solve our problems or ease our burdens.

In chiropractic this can often take the form of an obsession with adjusting technique. And while being able to reduce subluxations by restoring better spinal biomechanics is a valuable skill, a critical ingredient to successfully "delighting" patients is often overlooked: communication. In an effort to master the "art" of chiropractic, the patient often takes a back seat. "All I want to do is adjust," wails the doctor, frustrated by other responsibilities. All too many chiropractors would think they'd died and gone to heaven if they could somehow do nothing but silently adjust hundreds of patients each day. This technical aspect of chiropractic appeals to the shy, the introverted, and the self-esteem-impaired doctor.

This was an easy trap for many doctors to fall into during the exhilarating days of low insurance deductibles. Since chiropractic care intuitively feels good, and patients didn't have to directly "pay for it," doctors found patient compliance was practically automatic. In the early days, doctors could adjust and adjust and adjust for up to 30, 50, or more visits with little complaint from patients or insurance companies. It was an exciting time in chiropractic. If you missed it, ask some old-timers what it was like.

It's an understatement that things have changed. Doctors are recognizing that it takes more than delivering an excellent adjustment to get and keep patients. Doctors are recognizing it takes more than great results with a variety of symptomatic conditions to inspire and motivate patients to comply. Doctors are recognizing that a menu of creative (and legal) financial policies may be more important than the perfect admitting form, recall script, or adjusting table. Welcome to the future!

One solution is to become less adjustment-centered and more patient-centered. That doesn't mean delivering a slip-shod adjustment. It means that connected to the spine you want to correct is a cerebral cortex that requires the kind of adjustment that only superior patient communications can deliver.

When acknowledging that improving patient communications is needed, many doctors turn to *things*. Videos, brochures, posters, and other paraphernalia are made available to patients to fulfill this need. Yet, like the soldier and his light bulb, many doctors find that adding these tools does not automatically result in better educated patients. In the same way the soldier neglected the electrical generation plant, transmission wires, switches, and other infrastructure, doctors overlook their role in bringing these various tools to life. Success in breathing life into these "things" so they can "adjust" how patients think, is largely determined by how "internal" or "external" the doctor is.

The internal doctor is often self-conscious. Because he or she is careful to weigh all the facts before making any statement, and is so busy inside his or her head, they can often seem tentative, unsure, or distant to the patient. Patient conversations (when they occur) are more likely to revolve around the patient's technical improvement, rather than seemingly "less important" issues like the patient's work, family, or hobbies. When internal doctors speak, their pacing is slow, sometimes monotone, and their comments are often direct and to the point. While these doctors are often acknowledged to be excellent technicians, even winning awards in school, their practices are often low volume affairs that struggle from month to month.

The external doctor is gregarious, outgoing, and verbal. You always know where they are in the office because you can hear their booming voices or the delighted laughter of patients. They seem upbeat, optimistic, and engaging. They project their high energy level into everything they do. Oh, their desks may be a little sloppy and getting them to sit down to write a report can be difficult, but they have a loyal staff and patients. External doctors seem real and down to earth.

If the adjusting styles and patient recovery rates were identical, which doctor would have the larger practice? The external doctor, of course.

Unlike belly buttons, which some of us have "innies" and others have "outies," your personality and communication approach can change. If you recognize yourself as having more internal qualities than external, you can change. Because you've lived and reached your current level of success with your current communication style, shedding your internalism and becoming more external is going to feel uncomfortable and disorienting. In fact, your success to date will provide a strong pull *not* to change, which is why so few of us ever do. Most of us find a pattern of interacting with the world around us that gets us what we want, and we attempt to repeat this pattern indefinitely.

Think of coming out of your shell and being more external as learning and perfecting a new adjusting technique.

1. Sit in the front row. Most of the internal doctors I've met sit towards the back at seminars and other live presentations. They are practically voyeurs, barely participating in their own lives. These were the students who hoped the teacher wouldn't call on them in school. Today, their outlook is more that of a victim than a victor. And in a sense they *are* victims. They allow others to direct and control their lives. They have abdicated their responsibility to guide their destiny. Without a specific outcome in mind, they often just let life happen to themselves.

Put yourself in situations that can get you noticed. Just reading that sentence probably makes you nervous. I'm not suggesting showing off or strutting around the office like a peacock! Grab hold of life and participate.

2. Volunteer your opinion. The big lie internal doctors believe is the notion that the easiest way to skate through life and make sure everyone likes you, is to keep your opinions to yourself. When they express a point of view, it's likely *after* everyone else's so they can be sure it won't be controversial or politically incorrect. We often have the misguided notion that others will respect us more if we don't create waves or disagree. This attitude prevents many chiropractors from being articulate and outspoken chiropractic ambassadors.

While you may have become a master at hiding your tongue as you bite it, the internal battles raging in your mind can make you angry and bitter. Remember, it's just an opinion. Lighten up!

3. Take bigger risks. Start small. Maybe try some Thai food, take a different route to work, buy a "louder" necktie than you're accustomed to wearing. Listen to a different kind of music. Taking risks makes you stronger and more confident. It automatically forces you to take a proactive role in your life. Confront the fear that someone may find out by stepping outside the artificial barrier you've created for yourself.

Later, consider public speaking, taking post X-rays, or bungy cord jumping. Confront that which is holding you back, and it can no longer exert power or control over you. The only way out of bondage is to remove the spell it casts.

4. Reveal more about yourself. Since many of us who suffer from internalism often have a low self-image, sharing more about ourselves with others is difficult. Does anybody even care? Of course. Remember, the doctor role you play in our society can hinder others from getting involved with you. Besides volunteering your opinions, leave clues in your office via photographs or souvenirs about your hobbies, family, value system, community involvement, clubs, and other non-chiropractic activities. Provide a variety of entry points for others you encounter to engage you in conversation. You are an interesting individual (or you wouldn't have gotten involved in chiropractic) and your patients are curious and interested.

Thinking that you're strange, or don't fit in, or are somehow different or deficient just isn't true. Lead an open book life. Share your concerns, shortcomings, and dreams for the future.

Your vision may not be to see a hundred patients a day. That's fine. But remember, you have an important and honorable mission to accomplish in your community. The skills you possess are actually quite rare. You are the torchbearer of the truth that others went to jail to protect. The genealogy of your chiropractic ancestors were not those who were meek, apologetic, or lap dogs to anyone or anything! Reveal yourself. ■

TEN EXCUSES

When the stats are down or things aren't going right, the temptation is to look for someone or something to blame. Because few doctors look at their practices as a living organism, they often overlook the many organic causes of a drop off in new patients or other statistical areas of concerns. Instead, they make a trip out to the front desk.

True, the front desk staff member is the gatekeeper to the practice. Yet, that's not the first place to check. Look in the mirror. No one likes to accept the blame or the responsibility, but with all the finger pointing it's hard to know for sure. Until you know, you're likely to keep repeating the errors responsible for the new patient shortage.

If one's intelligence is measured by the ability to adapt to changes in the environment, today's doctor of chiropractic must be more intelligent than the one's twenty or thirty years ago. It is tempting to jump at the first right answer, embrace the opinions of seminar leaders, or to start doing what the doctor down the street is doing. These shortcuts for thinking for oneself overlook the fact that no one knows what the future will bring. Those that think they know, are simply good at extrapolating from current trends or just lying. Because no one knows that the future holds, we all have an equal chance to make accurate assumptions about it. The real issue is how much you trust your own instincts and how much confidence to have in yourself. Those with little of either are the most vulnerable.

Those quickest for blaming issues outside their control as the reason for their problems, regularly refer to certain factors. In no particular order, here's their top ten excuses:

1. Economy. This is a favorite among those who have difficulty communicating the value of chiropractic to their patients. Some doctors complain that the "recession" dropped their income as much as 20% last year. Others brag that it was their best year ever. It's not that the financial health of the country isn't a factor, it's how one deals with it. And simply claiming that you're "not going to participate in the recession" isn't the issue. You automatically participate if your patients or potential patients participate. What are you doing to adapt to the changing environment?

2. Weather. Snowstorms, hurricanes, tornadoes, flooding, a severe cold spell; like chiropractic and the Duracell bunny, the weather just keeps going. Few weather-related slowdowns last forever. But beating oneself up after a temporary downward blip in office statistics is crazy. If your office is healthy, like shedding wet clothes after a rainstorm, you should warm back up and be ready to pick up where you left off. If below the surface there is a fundamental lack of practice health with a reduced immune system response, weather could knock you out. But it's not the fault of the weather report!

3. Technique. Seems the grass is always greener on the other side of the fence. We learn about some doctor getting phenomenal results and the first question asked is what technique are they using. As doctors rush from one technique seminar to another, they become a "jack of all trades and a master of none." Besides the fact that most patients could care less what approach you use, clinical results would suggest that all the major techniques work. The key is mastering whatever technique that fits your individual physical and intellectual criteria. The goal is to achieve mastery without dogma. Make art.

4. Procedures. Finding the right office procedures by going from one management seminar to the next, successfully distracts some doctors for years. Thinking that finding and instituting a certain procedure will solve every problem, or worse, that once something works they won't have to ever change it again, plagues doctors who are destination or bottom line driven. Practice is a process. And the procedures that seem to work for thirty patients a day are rarely effective for sixty patients a day. The most adaptable doctors admit change is part of the agenda. Forever.

5. Competition. "Things would just be fine if the board wouldn't let all those new practitioners into the state," bemoans a doctor. "I remember when there were just the three of us in the whole town. Now there are over twenty chiropractors within five miles of my office," sniffs a 12-year veteran of practice. When the community sees a chiropractic office on every corner it can't help but raise the consciousness of the community and lead people to believe chiropractic is growing and becoming more successful. Hoarding a geographical area or adopting a scarcity outlook is counterproductive. Assure your right to survive by providing outstanding service, differentiation, clinical excellence, and exceeding patient expectations. It's called the free enterprise system. It's a wonderful example of homeostasis, benefiting patients and the doctors who serve the needs of their communities. If you've lost your unique factor or become irrelevant to the needs of your prospective patients, maybe the marketplace is trying to tell you something.

6. Insurance companies. The way some doctors talk you'd think the insurance industry was some type of private manna from heaven! What doctors weaned on $100 deductibles sometimes forget is that an insurance policy governs the relationship between the company and the patient. The health care service provider is just an unwelcomed fly in the ointment. The way some doctors are howling would lead you to believe that they feel they have some automatic claim, or that their patients deserve some type of special low deductible or carte blanche visit schedule when it comes to chiropractic. Dream on. If the changing insurance climate has changed your patient's ability to start, afford, or follow through with appropriate chiropractic care, what's your plan? It's likely to get worse. You'd have to think

Medicare was pure genus to hold out hope that the bureaucrats in Washington are going to save your practice.

7. HMOs and PPOs. Remember the cigarette advertising that featured smokers with fake black eyes stating they'd "rather fight than switch"? Many doctors are torn between the acceptance ("all my patients belong"), and the yoke of being told how long, how many, and how much. And for patients that look to a list for guidance in picking a doctor, it's a troublesome dilemma. More and more doctors are "getting on the list" and concentrating on the education of the patient so as to encourage a greater commitment to forms of continued wellness care not usually covered by managed care plans.

8. City. While the chamber of commerce of the town you're in would beg to differ, there really isn't a lot of difference between one town or another. Sure, the weather and geography may be different, but the patient attitudes, medical biases, and public perceptions about chiropractic are just about the same wherever you go. Thanks to the homogenizing affect of television, millions can see the CBS news story about chiropractic or read the *Wall Street Journal* article about chiropractic on the same day. The media makes a considerable impact on what people think and how they act. Whether they're told to "Nupe" their muscular aches and pains or that chiropractors are money hungry and are trying to seduce children into starting care, the media has a bias. But it's the same bias across the nation. It's not your city's fault that people don't seem to be available for chiropractic care.

9. Location. And within reason, it's not the fault of your office location that you're not getting enough new patients. Of course, if patients simply can't find a parking place or have to dodge crack cocaine dealers to get into your reception room, your location probably *is* a factor! Just remember, there was a time when people would fly from around the world to descend upon a little town in Wisconsin to get adjusted. If you have something people want and value, they will go to great lengths to get it. But if you've taken the path of least resistance and have been just peddling relief of neck and back pain, that may not be compelling enough to prompt patients to go to any extraordinary lengths to make appointments, keep appointments, or refer their friends and family. It's *not* your location.

10. I don't know. When a specific excuse isn't readily available, simply shielding oneself with a vague, "I-haven't-the-foggiest-notion" works perfectly. This one works the best because without being specific, there is little compulsion to investigate or take action steps to try to overcome the problem. It's a lot like when medical doctors can't seem to find the cause of the patient's problem they tell them "It's all in your head" or "You're just going to have to learn to live with it." Absolving any responsibility to try further, the M.D. simply throws up his hands, blames the patient, and gives up.

I've been in offices that by conventional wisdom shouldn't be seeing as many patients as they are. I've talked to doctors with poor grooming habits, lack detectable personalities, or muddle through with inadequate clinical skills, who enjoy enviable patient volumes. I've met staff members with attitudes that chase away patients, yet the practice continues to grow. I've had lunch with patients who know exactly what they'd do differently if it was their practice. The point is, there is a reason for everything. And anything can cause just about anything else. Focusing your examination on inside-out causes will almost always be more productive than looking for outside-in causes. It has a familiar ring to it and works great whether you're diagnosing a practice or a patient. ■

FIVE FEARS

About 50 years ago, in the depths of the Great Depression, president Franklin Roosevelt soothed a disoriented nation with his fireside chats. His reassuring sonorous tones and fatherly air of confidence were listened to with rapt attention. Many citizens felt despondent, fearful, and lacked confidence in the future. What Roosevelt did was reassure and provide direction. And while he set in motion many social programs and a dependence upon government that still burdens us today, the continuing loss of insurance coverage is causing a Great Depression among many chiropractors. Few are jumping from window ledges, but there are many who are questioning their commitment and future in this profession. Some have already left. And that's good.

Sadly, too many chiropractors got into the profession for the wrong reasons. Even today at chiropractic colleges, many instructors privately voice their alarm at how many students haven't even been adjusted until getting to school.

Not only did insurance "equality" open the doors to many patients who might not have tried chiropractic, it allowed doctors lacking poor communication skills or a chiropractic philosophy to survive, even thrive. Worse, dancing with the medically-oriented insurance industry fueled would-be medics interested in turning chiropractic into an extension of medicine. Witness the expeditions into manipulation under anesthesia, a desire to prescribe drugs, and those fighting to expand their state's definition of chiropractic to include breast and rectal examinations!

The more chiropractic becomes like medicine, the less attractive chiropractic will become.

The doctors I've talked to keep bumping up against five major fears facing their practices today. The good news is, with a little breathing into a paper bag to control the hyperventilation, there are some pretty simple solutions to a lot of them. As FDR said, "The only thing we have to fear, is fear itself."

1. Financial policies. Doctors who cut their teeth on $100 deductibles are finding more and more cash patients in front of them at the consultation and report of findings. The three-times-a-week-for-four-weeks-followed-by-two-times-a-week-for-four-weeks, etc. is increasingly being met by a distant stare. More and more patients aren't falling for the standard knee-jerk treatment schedule because of their financial condition. How many more patients do you have to put on some type of Financial Hardship Arrangement before you recognize that your hardship arrangement *is* your usual and customary fee?

Solution: Develop a menu of ways the patient can pay for their care. Consider a case fee and other arrangements that could make your care affordable for patients. Could your staff afford your typical initial intensive care recommendations if they weren't getting their care for free? Ask them. Create a variety of financial plans that work. Test them. Smell the coffee. Regardless of what Washington hatches for a nationalized health (sickness) plan, the 12 visits or so you may be granted won't save your practice. You must become more creative and resourceful and have many options at your disposal. The fees you'll be charging in the future will be a direct reflection of your ability to attach "value" to the care you're proposing for your patients. The more committed and communicative doctors will do just fine. Are you analytical, internal, and lack a terrific tableside manner? Shed the cocoon, procrastinate no longer, and get to a Toastmasters group! Your survival may depend upon it.

2. Reduced patient compliance and retention. This is related to the financial issue of attaching value to the care you're recommending. Unless you can attach enough value to the adjustment, patients become wary when a four minute procedure costs $35. Patients don't hang around for the 30-40 visits that insurance used to pay. Big problem.

Solution: Ultimately this is a communication problem. If you're still communicating the pinched nerve model of chiropractic instead of the more complete Vertebral Subluxation Complex approach, patients will continue to measure how they feel as a gauge for following your recommendations. You must explain the role of muscle and soft tissue involvement and the predisposition their long term neglect of their problem has for a relapse. If you don't, and patients drop out immediately upon getting symptomatic relief, when their problem returns, they will blame their poor judgment in consulting a chiropractor when their friends say, "I told you so." All things being equal, a patient's compliance is directly proportional to the rapport you're able to build, and your skills in explaining the chiropractic perspective to health and healing. Take a purely mechanical approach and use the superficial barometer of obvious subjective complaints as a guide, and no wonder the future seems frightening. Your view of chiropractic may be too small.

3. Reduced income and tighter cash flow. Nothing gets the palms more sweaty than when a doctor (or anyone else) finds their take home pay slipping while they are enjoying a lifestyle and overhead based on an insurance practice of the mid-1980s. Many doctors didn't recognize the trend until, after living off their receivables from huge personal injury cases of three or four years ago, their income plummeted.

Solution: At the root of most cash flow problems is the unwillingness to seriously question the overhead side of the ledger. Like the U.S. Congress that prefers to raise taxes instead of cutting waste and spending, many doctors look for ways to increase the income side of the equation. With this mindset, the notion of multi-level marketing of vitamins, soaps, and pure water devices actually starts looking attractive. Diversification is not the solution! If you'd put the time and energy into your practice that is spent opportunity chasing, your practice would generate much more cash, and the intangible thing we're all looking for: fulfillment. Concentrate on serving patients with 100% abandonment. Stop keeping score. Give. Remember, your paycheck is merely the result of the real or perceived value you're adding to the universe. Worrying about making the payroll or avoiding the confrontation of letting your unneeded staff person get on with his or her life is draining you of the energy and focus you should be giving your patients. The 1980s were great, but they're gone. Pick a convenient time and quickly go through the grieving process. Then, keep your eye on the ball and hunker down for the future. It's going to be fantastic.

4. Increased competition. "All the good spots for a chiropractic office are already taken," lamented a new graduate on the phone the other day. "A big HMO just moved into our town," groused a doctor at a seminar. "One of those chain clinics is starting up in our area, what should I do?" asked a doctor between short, shallow breaths. "The physical therapists are getting close to being permitted to do manipulation in our state..." There's plenty to worry about if you're one of those with a scarcity outlook on life (there's not enough patients to go around).

Solution: Doctors who were in practice before insurance equality, trust chiropractic and themselves enough to know that a chiropractor on every corner simply raises a community's consciousness about chiropractic. "Everybody seems to be doing it." Like those who single out immigrants as the cause for a lack of jobs, some are inclined to somehow limit the number of chiropractors in their state. The most fearful work their way onto the state board of examiners so they can more directly meter the number of newcomers. The cause of most scarcity outlooks is an unrecognized lack of confidence. Usually these are doctors who take things a bit too seriously and actually get their strength from seeing themselves as victims. These are the doctors out in the hallways at state conventions, gossiping and worrying about everyone else. Stick to your knitting. Make those doctors who are so threatening to you obsolete by making your own practice so compelling that no one would want to go to the "heathen" down the street. If you lack enough new patients, maybe you're the heathen!

5. Fear of the unknown. This is a time of tremendous change. The fear of the unknown that often prevents patients from seeking care, is holding back countless doctors. Some are holding out hope that some form of socialized health care is going to make the future bright. Others are wondering how the long term implications of the Mercy Conference document is going to impact them. The ambiguity of our times has normally competent doctors paralyzed with doubt.

Solution: Now, more than at any time since chiropractors were jailed for practicing medicine without a license, the profession needs doctors who are bold. The profession needs doctors who are proactive instead of reactive. This is when doctors must reaffirm their chiropractic philosophy and recall the "I'm-going-to-change-the-world" idealism that propelled them through cold winters in Davenport, or helped them endure months on four hours of sleep each night. The insurance era has bred a strain of doctors that may be too "accustomed to the smooth ride" as Paul Simon sang about in *The Rhythm of the Saints*. Take an inventory of all the "miracles" that you've facilitated. Count the number of patients' lives you've touched, changed, and enhanced. Rest assured of your future, knowing that if you can remain focused on serving your patients and adding value to their lives, your future is guaranteed.

The common denominator of these fears is the alarming trend by many doctors to look to outsiders for reassurance and confidence. Becoming dependent upon third party providers, whether government or industry, puts the doctor into bondage. Becoming dependent upon visionaries, whether management consultants or gurus, puts the doctor into slavery. Becoming dependent upon outside-in solutions fouls the fundamental connection with the forces that have permitted chiropractic to survive. Ignore, tamper with, or forget this cornerstone of chiropractic, and you will surely feel lost, isolated, and abandoned.

You are part of a great tradition that has weathered worse storms than this. Confront your fears and stare them down. After all, you created them. ■

THE PROBLEM
WITH MALL SHOWS

Many who profess to have the skills to help unlock the potential of private chiropractic practice seem to overlook a critical ingredient; the patient. For a profession that professes to look to the cause rather than to the treat symptoms, all too many of those rendering advice are overlooking the cause of many types of practice growth barriers. Putting an overemphasis on procedures, scripts, forms, and even the doctor's "headspace" ignores half of the success equation: the patient.

All too many management specialists either enjoyed their practice success at a different time in chiropractic (and with a different type of patient than today's image-conscious baby boom generation), or have such potent personalities that many of their suggested procedures are incongruent with the typical client doctor's personality. Focusing on the more visible and easily implemented internal tasks and paperwork is like medical researchers who study some narrow aspect of disease or physiology and ignore its interaction with the rest of the body. One day we hear coffee is bad, the next that it seems okay. Then it's bad. Then it's actually beneficial! Then it starts all over with decaffeinated coffee.

Any speaker, actor, or artist will tell you the audience is an important part of the performance. Ignoring the audience (patients) is a recipe for failure or risking the perception of indifference by the very people who write the doctor's paycheck. Relevance and sensitivity to the audience is critical.

That's why most chiropractic advertising is a waste of money.

Using advertising and other artificial stimulants to attract warm bodies with spines to an office is treating a symptom. Why don't current patients refer others? Why don't current patients continue with the same form of maintenance care that you enjoy, decreasing your need for more new patients? These questions get to the fundamental cause of a voracious appetite for new patients. The answers may not be pretty, but the truth should offer a practical game plan for the future.

"I'm either going to become a mall-show-new-patient whore or get an AK-47 and go berserk," said a doctor with quiet resolve on the phone the other day. Apparently he had just finished up with a consultant who had recommended an aggressive advertising program. In desperation he called to pick my brain.

"I'm just too good," he observed, revealing as much pride as frustration. "Patients come in here and they're feeling better in a couple of visits. It seems I get 'em well too fast and I have to keep looking for more new patients. So, what's the best type of handout for a mall show?" he asked, apparently not realizing he had abruptly changed the subject.

"Slow down," I interrupted. "One thing at a time. How often do *you* get adjusted," I asked.

"About once or twice a month," he answered cautiously.

"How come?"

"Just a habit I guess. Just to keep tuned up," he mumbled disinterestedly.

"Okay then, about how many adjustments does it take before your patient's start feeling better?" I asked.

"Usually about five or six," he said with his voice brightening.

"Why does it take more than one? The point is doctor, by the time most adult patients show up in your office there's been so much muscle and soft tissue damage that many will never really hold their adjustments and will need some type of on-going care for the rest of their lives."

"Yeah, that's probably true," he said.

"And when patients show up in your office, feel better, and

immediately discontinue care, how many are likely to have a relapse of their problem sometime in the future?" I asked.

"I don't know," he mumbled.

"Well, do you think 10% of your patients have their problem return?" I volunteered.

"Heck no, it's probably upwards of 80% to 90% I suppose."

"So what you're saying is that you've chosen to offer the easiest, most profitable, and least fulfilling type of chiropractic care?" I asked.

"I have patients who stay for thirty or forty visits or more!" his voice becoming more indignant.

"How do they pay for their care?" I asked.

"They're primarily work-related or personal injury cases," he admitted.

"So patients stay beyond five or six visits if they don't have to pay anything?"

The pause at the end of the phone made me wonder if he had hung up on me. Suspecting that the doctor was either having an "Ah-ha" experience or consulting the yellow pages for a gun shop, I waited.

"So what does that have to do with mall shows?" he said breaking the silence.

"Lots!" I said. "If you would educate your patients enough so that they would want at least the most minimal type of maintenance care you enjoy, you wouldn't need a constant stream of new patients. Plus, if you educated your patients better, they'd be better equipped to tell others about chiropractic, improving the referral process. Those are two immediate benefits of investing in better patient education."

I was on a roll now.

"Furthermore," I said, "patient education better assures that you'll be doing what a doctor should be doing, adjusting patients, not chasing patients down the mall with a plastic spine. It's not dignified, professional, and rarely attracts the types of patients you really enjoy serving!"

"But it's a good outreach for chiropractic," he countered.

"Different motive," I said. "If you can truly divorce yourself from the payoff of getting new patients for your investment of time and energy, knock yourself out. Because if your motive is pure; because the "little people" of the world need to know about chiropractic, that's different. But would you be willing to share the chiropractic gospel at a booth between Pet City and Music Land at the mall without the slightest chance of getting new patients?" I asked.

"Probably not."

Again I was greeted by a long silence. But this time I broke the quiet. "When you depend on advertising, free services, gimmicks, or other means to attract patients to your practice artificially, you're treating a symptom. The most efficient use of your energy is to uncover the cause of what's interfering with the natural referral process. You need to find out why your current and past patients aren't telling others. Until you know that..."

"I already know why," he said hastily, interrupting me.

"And what's that?"

"I'm not educating my patients," he said.

"So what are you going to do about that?" I asked.

"I'm going to do a mall show," as if his logic should be perfectly obvious to me.

It was then my turn to break the volley. During the silence I wondered what it really takes to change people. Is it something you say? Does all learning require the School of Hard Knocks? Did I just waste the last five minutes?

Like many doctors hooked on new patients with a pain relief only practice, stopping cold turkey is difficult. The temptation to do one more mailing, run one more ad, or try one more promotion is enticing. Secretly what these doctors know is that they've sold out. They took the path of least resistance, deferring to insurance company guidelines and living beyond their means as a compensation for low self-esteem. Now, the only thing they have to show for years of practice are countless X-ray files and artifacts of hundreds of brief patient encounters for headaches and low back pain. I'm not sure who was shortchanged more, the doctor or the patients. ∎

TAKING THE RISK

The seeds of failure are sown by the fruits of our success. All too often the procedures, sensitivities, and commitments we make that catapult us to success, are dropped when a certain level of "success" is reached. We buy more expensive homes, cars, and clothing to reflect our level of achievement. These trappings make it easy to lose touch with the habits and relentless pushing that led to our success. As we search for more comfort, more security, or the luxury we worked so hard to afford, we run the risk of becoming isolated in the corner office, protected by our loyal staff, and of delegating more and more of what we did that created our success.

Today, too many doctors are flabby and out of shape. This lack of conditioning is not necessarily a physical problem, but a mental dilemma. The days of an apparent endless source of new patients with $100 deductibles interfered with the sensibilities of even the most committed doctors. The personal relationships and tableside manners necessary to sustain long-term relationships with patients atrophied or never developed. The mutated strain of doctors emerging from the rollicking 1980s are entering a new era of chiropractic, like someone coming out of a darkened room and into the bright mid-day sun. Getting acclimated to this new environment will take more than rubbing your eyes and squinting for a few minutes!

Whether the old practice growing methods are beneath today's practitioner, seem "undoctorly," or require too much work, is hard to say. Ask any doctor if doing lay lectures and speaking to community groups would build their practice, and virtually all would agree it would. Ask any doctor if doing spinal care classes and new patient orientation talks would build their practice, and practically all would answer in the affirmative. Ask any doctor if calling every patient after their first adjustment would help solidify patient relationships and increase retention, and few would disagree. In fact, ask any doctor for a list of proven ways to grow a practice and all could supply an ample list–as long as they didn't have to actually *do* any of them!

Instead, we seem to prefer solutions that offer instant gratification. We gravitate towards the latest this or the newest that. We shy away from the tested and the proven. We seek out the high tech, push button, remote control way of getting new patients.

When all the smoke clears, there are only about seven sources of new patients. Which ones are you using?

1. Friends and family. This is where most new practitioners start. It is one of the biggest arguments for hanging out your shingle in your home town. Depending upon the size of your family and your social calendar, this is unlikely to generate the income that you dreamed about on those cold winter nights in school. Start here, but now what?

2. Advertising. This was unusually effective in enticing the least discerning types of patients into chiropractic offices in the 1980s when everyone had insurance. While this approach blackened the eye of the profession with unprofessional-looking (and sounding) advertisements, many practices attracted hundreds of people with spines into their offices. No matter that they didn't stay to benefit from maintenance care, the real money was extracted in the first thirty visits anyway. After the dust settled on all the "no out of pocket expense" offers, free spinal exam gimmicks, full page yellow page ads, and simplistic "bad back" oriented advertising lost its cost effectiveness, these same offices were left with valuable office space filled by patient files with brightly colored Avery labels. Patient education was ignored, administered haphazardly or inconsistently, so quality referrals weren't generated. Plus, the peer pressure on this image-conscious generation of patients prevented many from admitting to their friends that they had consulted an alternative, non-mainstream, charismatic huckster of a doctor who advertised on TV.

3. Referrals. Today, most practices depend upon satisfied patients who encourage others to seek care in the office they consult. It is the most effective, yet seemingly difficult way to attract new patients. By virtue of it's apparent uncontrollability, it is an important way prospective patients use to pick a health care professional. There are many ways offices can enhance the likelihood of the referral process happening such as exceeding expectations, patient education, improved accessibility, and low obligation entry points, among others. Since almost all of these approaches require more energy than simply making a biomechanical improvement in the patient's spine, they are largely overlooked by most doctors. A referral is not when you ask patients to supply the name of someone they know! That's something else.

4. Coercion. When patients are asked to betray a friendship and divulge a name, the doctor is exploiting his or position of power. While most patients resent this form of manipulation, it is still taught by some management groups as a legitimate way to build a practice! It's hard to measure how much damage this ploy has caused the profession, and how many patients reluctantly acquiesced through clenched teeth. Using this approach discourages long term patient relationships and thwarts the true referral process. Holding their X-rays hostage and demanding patients bring a friend to a group report is a related form of misuse of doctor power. Oh, it works, but at what cost?

5. Reactivations. While reactivations may not officially qualify as a "new" patient in the technical sense, many offices treat them as new patients statistically, so it should probably be mentioned here. For a patient to feel comfortable returning and perhaps risking an "I-told-you-so" attitude by the doctor or staff, is a remarkable accomplishment. It suggests that some form of patient education has been delivered and that patients weren't abused or chastised for not pre-

viously continuing with some form of maintenance care. Congratulations.

6. Mall shows. This is a special breed of new patient acquisition
that allows prospective patients to meet the doctor and sample his or
her bedside manner. Sometimes these are part of a "health fair," a
booth at a county fair, or folding table at a flea market. If it wasn't
for the environment, desperate attitude often projected by the doctor,
and "snake oil salesman" image that is often conveyed, it would be a
good approach. While getting out of the office and exposing the
doctor to the stupid questions, ignorance, and attitudes of the general
public can be a growth experience, it's a lot of work for the few
patients who follow through with their commitment. Funny, you
don't see too many dentists hawking at the mall. How come?

7. Public speaking. This is probably the most sophisticated and
effective way to plant new patient seeds. And while the instant
gratification of coupons and mailings are missing, it is a great way
to reveal your values, personality, and poise. Outreach programs, in
which you get to share your unique view of health and human
physiology, pay off by trusting the audience to do the right thing when
they feel it is appropriate. Honoring prospective patients in this way,
by avoiding incentives or gimmicks, attracts the most pleasant and
respectful patients. They are the type of patients you would most
enjoy serving. Too bad there are so few doctors who want to become
chiropractic ambassadors and take up public speaking.

No, after a few years of success as a processor of insurance
policies, too many doctors find that "getting their hands dirty" by
public speaking is just too much work. Never mind that for most
people public speaking is more terrifying than the specter of death.
Never mind that getting high quality new patients is almost guaranteed. Never mind that it is likely to be the only way unadulterated
chiropractic is ever going to get exposed to the general public. "Never
mind," doctors say, "what else do you have that I can use to get more
new patients?"

There are always other things doctors can do to get more new patients. But what is more interesting is the reluctance to confront this fear of public speaking. Virtually everyone knows that the rewards in business are almost always commensurate with the risk that is taken. The rewards of minimum wage workers are equal to the risk they take. The rewards enjoyed by entrepreneurs like a Bill Gates, a Ross Perot, or a Sam Walton are equal to the risks *they* take. Funny how we are so quick to avoid taking responsibility or risking our fragile self-esteems. More and more people seem to want governments, institutions, and corporations to take these risks for us. Just ask those recently laid off from some of the largest companies and outplaced from the military what security really is. It is in the ability to depend upon yourself. It is this attitude of self-reliance that built this nation and propelled covered wagons and mule trains across an inhospitable wilderness.

Only the strong will survive this insurance/health care/socialized medicine crisis. Those who are too lazy, too slow, or too fearful to claim their right to practice, will be forced to leave the profession or work for those with the tolerance to willingly assume the necessary risks. Join a Toastmasters group. Seek out opportunities to talk to others about chiropractic. Get out of your office. Become more accessible on the phone. Expose yourself to the real world. Take the risks now to develop the survival skills necessary to thrive in this new environment called the future. ■

THE PEACEABLE KINGDOM

As more and more chiropractic college students emerge from their studies with loans approaching six figures, and traditional health insurance continues to wane, new dangers are emerging for the direction of the profession. Some estimates suggest that more than 6,000 students are in school now, preparing to enter the marketplace. Some will make it. Others won't even try. And still others will try to find someone to work for. Philosophy? Who needs it? When you can smell the breath of your banker from over your shoulder, repaying the loan is paramount. So don't be surprised to learn that the future employer of many students will be a medical doctor.

Patients are going to love this arrangement. In fact, in many focus groups, patients express frustration with the battle lines that have been drawn between medicine and chiropractic. In their expedient desire for pain relief, what many patients want is medication for the short term combined with adjustments to address the real problem. If this could be conveniently offered at one location, many patients would be delighted. Chiropractors who think their patients are going home to empty their medicine cabinets after listening to an impassioned Wednesday evening health talk, are kidding themselves. Patients aren't willing to question the value of medications or dramatically change their behavior until chiropractic has clearly proven itself as a viable alternative—if then.

Some of the most aggressive and savvy medical doctors and HMOs have already recognized this. In these arrangements either chiropractors toe the line and get patients out the door in a minimum of visits, or they are no longer invited to participate. In an effort to "play the game" many chiropractors have become biomechanical pain relief agents, and the notion of wellness or maintenance care for their patients has atrophied. The graduate who dreamed of changing the world has become a spine mechanic.

It's interesting how so many chiropractors want to be accepted, even embraced by the medical community. Many have this idealistic vision of working side by side medical practitioners in a "Peaceable Kingdom" arrangement in which hospital privileges are just the beginning. Some of the most articulate chiropractors jump at occasions to argue the case for chiropractic at local medical society meetings or debates sponsored by the local public television station. What these chiropractors are missing in their quest to prove the correctness of chiropractic, are the ramifications of actually winning the debate!

"The fact is ladies and gentlemen, what my medical friend has overlooked is that structure and function are related, and normalizing spinal function helps normalize nervous system function. Cutting out parts, using drugs to slow down or speed up gall bladders or digestion, without first normalizing structure, borders on insanity and harbors a gross disrespect for the patient."

The audience looks in stunned horror as the medical doctor leans on the podium and puts his head in hands. Suddenly he looks up, and with confidence he addresses the television audience.

"My chiropractic colleague is absolutely correct. In fact, I have known this myself for the last two years, during which time I have investigated chiropractic and have learned these tested spinal adjusting approaches from some of the best chiropractors in the country. And I am here this evening to announce a shift in my own practice that will incorporate chiropractic, backed up by my own 15 years of experience as a medical doctor..."

Farfetched? Not really. What many chiropractors overlook is that given the choice between conservative chiropractic care from a chiropractor or a medical doctor, a huge majority of the public would first consult the medical doctor. The fact that you believe your adjusting skills are better than a couple of weekend courses attended by the opened-mined-market-sensitive medical doctor, would have little bearing on the actions of the general public.

If you do a really good job of convincing the medical community how effective chiropractic is, many might decide to add chiropractic techniques to their little black bag of tricks.

Don't worry. They're not going to waste their time learning how to adjust. Instead, it will be far easier to employ hungry new graduates fresh out of school. If you thought being an associate doctor for a chiropractor was pharaoh-like bondage, wait until you see what entrepreneurial medics might have up their sleeves. It won't be pretty.

This won't be a philosophical skirmish or even a tacit admittance that chiropractic is better. It will be purely a financial transaction. Those with financial resources always control those without. With chiropractic philosophy missing from most schools these days, the decision between the ability to pay back school loans by being an employee of a medical doctor, versus the more challenging fears of starting up one's own practice, will be an easy choice for all too many.

The key issue here is that being an employee of a medical doctor is not the same as being an employee of a chiropractic doctor, even if the pay were identical. The dues-paying process sounds similar, but it's not. Unlike being a chiropractic associate in a chiropractic office with the opportunity to have one's own patients, and being continually "fed" in the chiropractic tradition, the only mentor the new chiropractic graduate has in the medical doctor's office will be the medical doctor.

You've probably seen the nature films on television in which the mother chicken adopts a baby goose that has been abandoned or a cow accepts a baby goat as her own. The problem is, the goose starts thinking it's a chicken and the goat a cow. Same problem here. The student is barely able to pay off his or her student loan, but starts thinking like a medical doctor. Shunned by the medical community and distrusted by his chiropractic colleagues, he becomes a mixed breed, lacking focus, direction, and a clear identity.

The future of chiropractic, not only legally, but philosophically, is better assured by being different from the medical community. If the lines ever get blurred by the public, chiropractic (like osteopathy) will be the loser. However, to the new graduate struggling to find a way to pay back the bank, the issue will be personal survival, not professional purity. What these new graduates will learn the hard way is that the "patients" they get will be the ones discarded by the medical doctor. Without an identity, the new graduate will make enough money to make loan payments and barely get by. Years later he or she will still be in bondage, merely making payments. They will be doing themselves a disservice by prolonging the inevitable: biting the bullet and trusting themselves.

If you don't feel like you have the personality, energy, or adjusting skills to go it alone, at least work with a chiropractor! But if you must sell your skills on the open market, recognize you will have to do the same thing the impoverished immigrant must do to escape the poverty of the ghetto: save. "But everything is going to pay the bills, there's nothing left over to save," I can hear you say. Move to a less expensive home or apartment. Drive a less expensive car. Don't eat out. Too much sacrifice? Then buy some lottery tickets instead. For some reason, all too many graduates think they somehow *deserve* their career. Many can't understand why they're not driving big cars home from their offices to estates after just a year or so of practice.

For some, this shock of reality will be too much. It will chase some into the grasp of medical doctors, HMOs, or some type of "therapist" position somewhere else. And the so-called progress that has been made in the last hundred years; the jailed chiropractors, the research, the chiropractic pioneers, and the miracles, will have been in vain.

Remember this the next time you want to be "accepted." Why did you choose chiropractic anyway? ■

THE BUDDY SYSTEM

The continued attraction of chiropractic seminars, management groups, and conventions is evidence that there is an apparent need to be in contact with other doctors. Perhaps this is because doctors work mostly by themselves, isolated from other practitioners, and have few opportunities to share ideas or discuss concerns with intellectual peers. While some of the most secure doctors have surrounded themselves with bright staff members who can partially serve in this capacity, an employee relationship often precludes discussing certain issues or revealing fears, shortcomings, or strategic business decisions. Lacking this support structure, doctors may be tempted to choose certain patients to confide in, or succumb to buying this kind of relationship from an agenda-laden management firm.

An individual or group with the wrong motives can exploit the confidences that are naturally shared in this context. Subtle forms of manipulation ("You can't do it alone these days...") or self-serving sales messages ("Increase your billings with our XYZ machine...") can cloud the distinction between coaching and copulation.

What many doctors want is some type of mentoring relationship. Those that pay for management counsel are often those who willingly admit they lack the discipline, courage, or experience to successfully run the business part of their practices. Most are happy with their clinical skills and have practices of delighted patients. And while treating the most obvious needs of paperwork systems, staff hiring, and business management can produce bottom line improvement, the underlying problems of personality, fear, courage, vision, responsibility, communication, and other very personal issues are often ignored or conveniently overlooked. These fundamental concerns are difficult to modify during superficial telephone exchanges or ballroom-sized pep rallies. This is largely due to the consultant's notion that becoming vulnerable and revealing his or her own shortcomings would be unprofessional and counterproductive. Yet, consultants who are confident and recognize that they don't have to have the right answers all the time, are more likely to foster an atmosphere of mutual trust in which personal issues can be broached. There are other ways of building trust than simply supplying advice that increases a doctor's take home pay!

I got a letter from an especially resourceful chiropractic student who recognized the value of surrounding himself with good advisors and having mentors to consult. He wrote me requesting a list of the doctors who had influenced me, so he could secure them as mentors too. While I was flattered that he was seemingly interested in emulating my world view by reading my books and hunting down those who had shaped my outlook, I had to deny his request. You don't create a mentorship armed with a typewriter and a mailing list.

A mentor relationship contains certain key elements:

Win/win: What is often overlooked is that the best mentor relationships are win/win in nature. Both parties must benefit in some way, or there is little incentive to continue. But what can an experienced veteran doctor get out of a mentorship with a twelfth quarter student? The student can gain wisdom and insight, and the veteran field doctor can experience the joy of sharing, teaching, and leading. It is not unlike the role of father and son; mother and daughter. When this hard to measure equilibrium is out of balance, the relationship ends. Those you seek as mentors must perceive some form of benefit from the exchange, or it will not develop.

No financial gain: Mentors do not exchange money or charge for the contributions they make to each other. It is common for both parties to benefit financially and otherwise from the relationship, but not directly. The lack of financial return often thwarts established groups from setting up "mastermind" and other ad hoc groups that can serve to brew these types of valuable mentoring opportunities. Like oil companies that are accused of dragging their feet in developing solar energy technologies because they "can't find a way to tax the sun," there are built in deterrents to actually discourage these types of relationships.

Mutual trust: Trust is a fundamental building block to mentorship. It requires a level of intellectual, spiritual, and emotional intimacy that may be uncomfortable for some. Certainly it means shared values and vision. Age may not be a factor so much as an openness and nonjudgmental communication style. Without a mutual respect, you have superficial conversations in which few of the risks necessary for personal breakthroughs can occur. In a mentor relationship there is little room for those who perceive themselves as victims or carry the burden of enlarged egos.

Similar values: This is the touchstone that not only defines the possibility of mentorship taking roots, but predicts whether the relationship will bloom. A shared vision for chiropractic, a congruent approach to spiritual issues, a similar appreciation for esthetics, a sensitivity to time, even attitudes about money, form a mosaic that another may or may not find intriguing. When enough of these values are shared, the likelihood of mentorship growing into a mutually rewarding relationship is high.

If it were my objective to facilitate a doctor's acquisition of a mentor, I would send him or her a simple questionnaire. Besides asking the obvious like name, address, age, marital status, schooling, adjusting techniques, political orientation, years in practice, practice volume, and the like, I'd ask questions about their religious and worship involvement, hobbies, whether they make decisions based on facts or feelings, whether they have connections to other cities or parts of the country, areas of their practice that they feel weak and strong, and other specifics that could reveal one's attitude and personality. Returning this questionnaire along with a nominal "finders fee," and the information would be put into some type of matchmaker type database program. The objective wouldn't be to find perfect matches, but to find like-mined individuals who would have the likelihood of "hitting it off."

My mentors are spread all across North America. The trouble with trying to find a mentor in your town, is that many might find that too competitive. It might be better that at least a couple hundred miles separate both doctors. Let's say you practice in Dallas and maybe you have relatives in the Boise area. Great, let's find a compatible doctor interested in this type of program in the Boise area and introduce the two of you. Or maybe you're a devout Catholic and you're looking for encouragement from another like-minded chiropractor. Or perhaps you're more analytical and recognize the need to enhance the expressive side of your personality. I believe there is someone out there, maybe on the other side of the country that would like to pick your brain and get to know you better.

I contend that deep down, just about every doctor knows what he or she needs to do to improve his or her life and practice. The challenge is to find someone who can provide the rapport, encouragement, and safety net in which new ideas can be tried. It may not be necessary to turn to an official consultant. In fact, if anything, many of the issues that need to be addressed to free up the growth of a practice would be better handled by a psychologist, therapist, church leader, or other non-chiropractic specialist. The problem is rarely chiropractic in nature. It's just the arena in which the problem is revealed.

After awhile, those fortunate enough to have a well established network of mentors, discover that an amazing thing happens. When you're basking in the success of a "win," you know just who to call to offer a friendly kick in the pants. And the reverse happens. It seems someone knows just when you could use some encouragement to brighten your day, and they call you. It's rarely planned. It just happens that way. Part of the joy of participating in a mentoring relationship is using your sixth sense to know when to call and catch up on things.

What do mentors talk about? Sure, some of it is gossip. Some of it is problem solving. But a lot of it is sharing ideas and perspectives. These conversations serve as a way to process events and help give meaning to one's experiences. Things that may seem threatening or significant in some way to you, can be viewed by another with an entirely different interpretation. This pooled brainpower can broaden your perspective and help you respond more confidently and re-sourcefully to the challenges around you.

This buddy system is something that swimmers, skin divers, skydivers, rock climbers, and others engaged in dangerous or exotic activities use to help protect, support, and encourage each other. In today's fast changing practice climate, what could be more exotic and dangerous than practicing chiropractic without a mentor? ■

THE BIGOTRY OF BIG

We start comparing ourselves with others at an early age. Even as early as junior high school when we start communal showering after physical education class, our furtive glances and stolen glimpses are used to compare them with us. "Am I normal?" becomes an unspoken mantra through high school as we try to fit in. Later in life, keeping up with the Joneses and all the other peer pressure that makes it difficult to be an individual, is practically taken for granted. "What will the neighbors think?"

Our self esteem is a major indicator of how much influence others will wield in our lives. When our self image is low, we are susceptible to all kinds of ideas and are willing to embrace the behavior of the dominant influencing group in our life. How else can you explain cigarette smoking, male earrings, lime green leisure suits, and other actions that sabotage our health, display our poor judgment, or label us as eccentrics?

Since you chose chiropractic, you are one of the true individualists. You seek the truth, even if it goes against the grain. You embrace a profession that conventional wisdom tells us doesn't work, isn't needed, and is used as a last resort. You may even have relatives that scorn you for your career choice and don't understand your purpose and vision. When you can't even get blood relatives to accept chiropractic, it's no wonder you have problems with the skeptical patients who show up in your consultation room!

You're a Lone Ranger. You're willing to stand up for the truth.

You know that when millions of people "believe" in a bad idea, it's *still* a bad idea. I congratulate you on your commitment.

But there's this little problem with practitioners who have larger practices than you. You know the ones. The ones who may only spend a few minutes with their patients. The ones who couldn't possibly be rendering optimum patient care. Your reaction to these doctors, their procedures, and their practices tells a lot about you.

Are you a bigot?

Automatically thinking large volume practitioners are providing slipshod care, are only in it for the money, or must be doing something illegal, immoral, or unethical, are the same type of knee jerk reactions you see in racists. Most of these generalizations and characterizations of high volume practitioners are simply wrong. Ignoring them, spreading rumors, secretly hoping for their failure, or smugly knowing that your style of practice is *the* correct one, are probably some of the very reasons your practice isn't having the influence in your community that theirs are. Ironic, isn't it?

Today, a high volume practice is the best "insurance policy" for the uncertainty that plagues the health care profession. It's the same form of insurance that served chiropractic doctors of the 1960s, 1970s and before. Offices that have patient volumes in the range of a hundred patients a day or more are considerably less concerned about these volatile times than offices struggling to see twenty or thirty patients a day.

Would you accuse Dr. Clarence Gonstead of having provided slipshod care or of having done something illegal? Or Dr. Clay Thompson? Dr. Joseph Janse? Or any of the other leaders in the profession before insurance equality?

Of course not.

While it's a great defense mechanism to rationalize that anyone with a larger practice than you must be doing something sneaky or tricky, that's rarely the case. Are there large practitioners that bend the rules and get certified letters from the state board of examiners?

Of course. The fact is, when you're a "big gun" you're constantly under a microscope. Do something illegal and you don't last.

This is not to suggest that a large practice is somehow better or that doctors who prefer a more "boutique" approach to their practice are inferior. It is merely to suggest that large practitioners are making a significant impact in their communities. Since few doctors I meet wish to stay at their current size, perhaps incorporating some of the approaches used by busier offices could help. Here are few to try on for size:

It's a business first: Large practitioners don't look at it that coldly, but the cold hard facts are that if you can't deliver, charge, and collect more for your adjustments than it costs you, they don't let you help others very long. Staff members demand pay and the landlord demands rent. You may have stumbled upon the healing secret of the ages, but if you can't exchange your services in such a way that you end up with more money than you pay others, your influence will be minimal.

Systematized infrastructure: High volume offices are made possible by creating and maintaining a *system* of serving their patients. This system reduces confusion, empowers staff members to act appropriately, and frees the doctor from routine and mundane decisions. Not only does this allow the doctor to focus on seeing patients, it leverages his or her talent so that more patients can be helped. When mistakes or errors occur, flaws in the system are blamed, not the staff. Teamwork and cooperation flourish.

Talented delegators: These doctors know that they cannot do everything themselves. They have developed the skills (it is a learned behavior) to empower, inspire, and lead their staff. The same ability to plan, implement, and communicate a way of doing business, is the same ability needed to direct patients. In short, they know how to get things done through others. They are "doers" and can hold a clear image in their minds of the outcomes they want for as long as it takes.

Sell talent not time: Doctors who see a lot of patients each day make sure their patients understand that they are buying the doctor's talent, not his or her time. The only way to spend three minutes with a patient and motivate him or her to willingly return for future visits, is to communicate the value of the adjustment, not by selling a ten or fifteen minute experience with the doctor!

Incredible focus: Regardless of the school they graduated from or their adjusting approach, high volume practitioners are extremely focused. They are not easily swayed by the fads and gimmicks that come and go in the profession. They do not attend every seminar that springs up and fades out. It's not that they reject new ideas or are unwilling to try new things. It's that they know that the fundamentals of helping lots of people and running an effective organization depend upon issues such as honesty, fairness, exceeding patient expectations, love, service, and other topics that rarely show up at weekend seminars. They stay on purpose by not allowing the purpose of others to distract them.

Have a big vision: Like other leaders in the profession, these practitioners have big dreams for their practices and their patients. Because they have an abundance outlook on life, knowing that there are more than enough patients to go around, they are unafraid of a few patients not liking what they do. They are unconcerned about other doctors "stealing" their patients. Patients respect and admire their focus and determination. Patients recognize they are being seen by a doctor whose influence and reach is beyond the three to five mile radius enjoyed by ordinary offices.

Outgoing personality: Every high volume practitioner I've met shares this apparent critical aspect. I'm sure there are exceptions, but a large practice demands an incredible communicator at the helm. Thousands of less influential doctors already recognize superb clinical skills and stunning results don't automatically result in a huge practice. This frustrates many who find the technical aspect of delivering the adjustment the most pleasurable part of practice. Ironically, it is one of the least important when it comes to attracting and keeping large numbers of delighted patients. This isn't to downplay the importance of the adjustment, it's just that patients expect results. Delighted patients, referrals, and productive long term relationships result from clearly communicated compassion, involvement, and exceeding each patient's expectations. That requires the sensitivity to be a good listener and the self-confidence to risk revealing yourself.

Give more than you take: This may be the hardest for struggling doctors to appreciate or accept. Most large volume practitioners give more than they take. They are always reinvesting back into their patients and their practices. The fundamental laws of the universe are centered around service to others. This isn't giving to get! This is the logical response of a true servant attitude. It is the natural reflex of recognizing one's debt to others for having learned valuable healing skills to share with the world. This humbling spirit keeps doctors in touch with God and brings balance to their worldly achievements.

These are just a few of the characteristics I have seen in the offices with high patient volumes. Notice that the word "success" doesn't appear once. Having a large practice is not how success is defined in chiropractic! Having a million dollars in tax-free municipal bonds is not necessarily success. Having the expensive house, flashy jewelry, or other ostentatious displays is not true success either. How do *you* define success? ■

PATTERN RECOGNITION

I remember Eric coming home from second grade one day, proudly reporting that he was good at finding patterns. "What do you mean?" I asked. "The teacher said I was good at finding repeats," he said earnestly. "I can tell what's coming next by looking at what comes first." He instantly changed the subject, not knowing the significance of his discovery, or how it would serve, or plague him in the years ahead. In fact, some would say that most of us spend the rest of our lives trying to find "repeats."

Pattern recognition is a major part of our education. Perhaps at first, the patterns are no more than telling light from dark, moving shapes from stationary objects. Over the years, like an obedient dog at Pavlov's beck and call, we learn to associate certain sounds with words, certain words with their meanings, and so it goes until we have a vocabulary. This process repeats itself in many other ways until we have a model that describes the actions and reactions of the world around us. Slowly we learn to predict the outcomes of conversations, based on our ability to recognize patterns of human interaction. We're able to predict the outcomes of television shows based on our ability to recognize patterns in plot development. And so it goes, until we feel like we have pretty much mastered our world. If we limit our exposure to the world, we need only recognize a relatively small number of patterns to survive. Enter into the world of politics, commodity futures, international finance, or health care, and the patterns are more varied and complex.

For the same reason we study history, a major advantage of good pattern recognition skills is the ability to avoid mistakes and better predict the outcomes of situations around us. The desire to control our destiny by accurately predicting the results of our actions and those of others can be quite appealing. Those who discover successful patterns of patient acquisition, patient care, and patient retention are inclined to repeat these patterns again and again.

Yet, dependence upon these success patterns is a double-edged sword. The same skill we use to get the results we want, puts us in a rut. At first, predictable outcomes provide security and allow us to direct our energies to more pressing needs. Later, we can feel oppressed and bored. When we discover the "formula" for success, it can make practice uninteresting.

The most alarming, of course, is when we learn a pattern that creates the outcome we want, begin depending upon the pattern, and then suddenly find the outcome changes. Suddenly, we discover patients don't do what "they're supposed to do" based upon our outdated model. This is what more and more doctors are discovering.

It used to be getting new patients from a lay lecture was a slam-dunk. It used to be getting new patients from yellow page advertising was a sure thing. It used to be patients would stay for the full course of treatment. Whether the "patterns" doctors were depending upon were a scripted recall program, a canned report of findings, or some other proven procedure that resulted in predictable patient behavior, much has changed. This must be unsettling for doctors who never really "owned" the procedures, scripts, or chiropractic, for that matter.

What more and more doctors are recognizing is that the tried and true scripts from the past aren't working like they used to. This is largely because today's practice environment has changed. The financial aspects of care have become huge barriers for doctors accustomed to having their recommendations automatically accepted by patients because they were covered by insurance. Insurance equality created a mutated strain of chiropractor unable to cope with the practice realities of the 1990s. Weakened by low deductibles, corrupted by high fees, and tempted by easy money from unattended therapies, many of today's chiropractors are searching for new patterns.

There are patterns! While many will cling to the past, try to ignore the new realities, or even deny things have changed, the survivors will be the ones willing to recognize and adapt to these new patterns. Many doctors have already acknowledged these new patterns and have developed appropriate procedures. Here, in no particular order, are a few worth considering:

Separating cost from care: With ample insurance money and low deductibles, it was easy for many doctors to ignore the financial implications of their care recommendations. Just about anyone could handle the low deductibles, so the purpose of the report of findings was to outline an optimum treatment program of thirty, forty, or more visits. Few doctors ever had to say that "...each adjustment I render will cost $___." Well trained staff members avoided the embarrassment and doctors could remain "pure" and detached from the financial realities.

Predetermined budget: While patients won't tell you this, many enter your office with a price in mind, of what they're willing to pay to recover. Since the lack of insurance or a high deductible automatically makes them a cash patient, they have a number in mind before entering your office. Whether this figure is $100, $250, or $500 is a well-guarded patient secret. Some might claim that incredible patient education can help raise this number, and I'd agree. The point is, you can use up this "budget" with an expensive exam, X-rays, and a few visits, and risk patients thinking chiropractic doesn't work. Or, recognizing this, you can structure your fees to permit more visits, enhancing the patient's perception of the value of chiropractic care.

Financial policy menu: While on the subject of money, you will need to become much more resourceful by offering patients many different types of choices for paying for their care. Case management fees, "you-buy-eight-and-we'll-give-you-ten," and other creative approaches have become necessary. The real challenge is keeping your "usual and customary" fees high for those occasional personal injury cases, while making it affordable for your cash-paying patients. Serving two masters isn't possible, and "leaving money on the table" on those juicy personal injury cases runs counter to the financial insecurity many doctors are feeling these days. Pick one.

Quality is paramount: The free spinal exam and all the other gimmicks of the past are counterproductive. More and more of the decision-makers shaping the direction of health care reform find that these marketing ploys devalue chiropractic. Quality, in everything from business cards and office decor to phone skills and tableside manners, is critical. Patients don't want the cheapest care, they want the best. How are you projecting quality and attention to details in your office?

Increasing accountability: Many have already discovered this, but the trend for the future is more reports, more second-guessing by "authorities," and the need for excellent patient records. Documentation, while not the glamorous part of patient care, is becoming more and more important. If you're not keeping SOAP notes with every patient, get started.

Over communicate: Medical doctors already recognize that chiropractic doctors have a huge head start in this area. Patient communication skills will become increasingly important as patients must reach for their own wallet to pay for their care. Remember, patients do what they do, because they think what they think. Changing the way patients think is an every-visit responsibility of doctor and staff. Symptomatic improvement may "buy" the patient's body, but patient education "buys" the patient's mind–controlling compliance and retention.

Low commitment entry points: Because of the new financial realities and the myth that "once you start seeing a chiropractor you have to go for the rest of your life," new ways of introducing patients to chiropractic need to be considered. Actually showing up in your office is a huge commitment for many, so it is often delayed as long as possible. Create an information packet about chiropractic and advertise its availability among your current patients. Invite no-obligation office tours. Collect the names of satisfied patients willing to put prospective patients at ease about your office and your procedures. Invite prospective patients to call and ask questions anonymously over the phone. Create ways potential patients can get their "feet wet" before plunging in.

Reduced overhead: This is a biggie. More and more offices are discovering that they no longer require thousands of square feet of office space. More doctors are waking up to the realities that they are overstaffed. While it's difficult to say goodbye to a trusted staff person, a top-heavy overhead structure is inappropriate in today's marketplace. Take a hard look at what you need to provide quality care. Do you really need someone to escort the patient and their travel card down the hall? Would a part-time person work out better than a full? Do you really need two people at the front desk? Question the status quo.

Recognizing new patterns and developing appropriate responses to them is a new skill for many. Simply doing more of what used to work isn't the solution either! And while scripted responses to the world around us offer a sense of security, all too often they obscure procedures or manipulative schemes that are no longer in touch with the times. Pattern recognition is a major part of the diagnostic process with patients, or your practice. How good are your pattern recognition skills when it comes to diagnosing what ails your practice? ∎

RUSH HOUR DOGMA

One of my favorite moments of Lucille Ball's tremendous television career was the cake assembly line sketch. Lucy and Ethel were given the job of putting cherries on the tops of frosted cakes and then putting the finished cakes into boxes. At first the assembly line moved at a modest pace, making it possible to easily complete the task. The laughs started as the conveyor belt increased its speed and Lucy and her accomplice couldn't keep up. And while few doctors and their staff find it an occasion to laugh, a similar phenomena occurs in many offices during the rush hour each evening. In a silent version of musical chairs, patients seek a finite number of appointment "slots" with the shortest wait. Doctors lament over the lost revenue of patients who decide that their symptoms don't justify the wait. Staff members bemoan the daily tally of no shows. And some patients resent the apparent popularity of their doctor. Mastering the peak times of the day and maximizing its productivity separate the struggling doctor from the successful doctor.

In established offices the patient volume seen between about 4:30 PM and about 6:30 PM is an important indicator. The staff's efficiency is demonstrated during this 2-hour period, and so is the doctor's philosophy, self-image, and ability to recognize the essentials of doctoring.

The ability to master the hours of peak demand dictate the impact your office will have in your community. To increase your patient volume during this critical time of the day when everyone wants to receive care, will almost always require some type of change.

Whether this change is attitudinal or procedural, it will feel uncomfortable at first. In fact, changes that are needed may be so unsettling they may preclude any change at all, enshrining the status quo. While that's every doctor's right, it's always a shame to see opportunity squandered and the responsibility to help others thwarted unnecessarily. Which one of these suggestions makes you the most uncomfortable?

Selling your talent not your time: It still amazes me how many doctors feel obligated to spend two or three times as much time adjusting a patient than it takes to adjust their spouse. It's clearly not a clinical issue—no one would give their spouse substandard care! "My patients expect at least a 10 minute adjustment for $XX!" Who gave the patient that expectation? "The other chiropractor spent XX minutes so they want me to spend that much time too," shrugs a doctor. So now we're allowing the slowest, least-confident doctors in the profession to set the pace? "I don't feel like I'm being thorough enough if I take less time," says another doctor in a holier-than-thou tone of voice. Interestingly, these are the same doctors who "buy into" the patient's symptoms and are less likely to trust the patient's own inborn healing ability. If a doctor assumes too much responsibility for the patient's recovery, this time trap is an easy one to fall victim to. Make sure each patient understands that for the cost of the adjustment they are buying your *talent* and not your time. It takes much less time for an experienced carpenter to build a house than a union apprentice. Make sure patients know they're actually buying years of schooling, the experience of delivering thousands (maybe millions) of adjustments, and the expertise of a frequent seminar-goer and a voracious journal reader. Communicate these concepts to every new patient. Still comfortable? Then continue...

Use a faster technique: Since this profession is so dogmatic about technique, this suggestion usually does little more than make the hairs on many doctors' backs bristle. But here goes anyway. As someone who hasn't been to technique seminars or been given the "what-ever-you-do-don't-allow-anyone-to-adjust-you-using-the

XYZ-technique" speech, I'm not sure I fully understand all the commotion. The fact is, virtually all the techniques floating around these days work. I've been adjusted with the top dozen or so approaches and found them all effective. Those who squander precious moments with esoteric diagnostics, involved muscle testing, and other time-consuming preambulary procedures, seem to gain confidence and a sense of self-righteousness from their uniqueness. Ironically, these procedures, often performed in complete silence, do little to build a patient's sense of confidence in the doctor. If the excellent clinical results high volume practitioners achieve is any indication, this is a time-consuming form of ego gratification that can waste valuable time during the peak hours of demand. Find a faster technique. Countless doctors who employ approaches that more quickly restore improved motion along fixated joint planes get excellent results. Today's busy patient appreciates the short office visit and the confidence projected by a "let's-get-to-the-point" office visit. Reducing the visit to the essentials of restoring better biomechanics helps patients assume the proper perspective about their chiropractic care. Patients need to know the most valuable part of their visit is the adjustment, not the therapy, not the diagnostics, not the magazine reading, or the other procedures.

Use fewer adjusting rooms: It doesn't take a time and motion expert to determine that when you're opening and closing doors and walking (even a few short steps) down the hallway, it's not a productive use of your expertise. While at first glance "storing" patients in three or four adjusting rooms seems to make sense, it wastes precious seconds. And that's how improved rush hour productivity is measured—in seconds. Using a single adjusting room with an "on deck" chair or two just outside the room can be very efficient. Similarly, two tables six or seven feet apart and only separated visually by a wall divider can improve capacity. Many doctors avoid this capacity enhancing arrangement because they think patients will complain about the lack of conversational privacy. And it's true, at first they may. But as long as you point out the closed door of your office across the hall, and your willingness to discuss private matters at their request, it shouldn't be a problem. In fact, it will keep you and the patients focused on their purpose for being in your office! It's not to discuss the ball scores or conduct some complimentary psychological counseling! "Oh, but it seems like an assembly line," I can almost hear you say. And you're absolutely right. The question is, are you turning out X widgets an hour or XX widgets? Going slower by increasing the physical distance between patients doesn't change anything except your capacity. And most patients, especially if you tell them, will appreciate the opportunity to get in and get out of your office quickly so they can get on with their lives. Still with me? Try the next one on for size.

Streamline your procedures: An old family recipe for baked ham was handed down from generation to generation. The first instruction was to cut 2" off one end of the ham. For years this direction was followed without question. When the recipe was turned over to the newest member of the family, she asked why the 2" was to be cut off. Was it to add flavor? Did it reduce the cooking time? What was the purpose? It wasn't until the surviving matriarch of the family was consulted, that the answer was revealed. "My cooking pan wasn't big enough so I always had to cut 2" off," came the matter of fact answer. How many of your current procedures, begun years ago at a lower office volume, no longer serve you? Maybe all you need to do to increase your productivity is to buy a bigger pan! Is it time for a better adjusting table? Is it time to stop wasting valuable seconds giving patients a ride on your adjusting table? Is it time to revise your travel cards and other paperwork for better efficiency? Is it time to discontinue having staff members escort patients down the hall? Are there portions of the new patient procedure or aspects of the report of findings that can be delegated to other staff members? What's adding extra steps, wasted motion, or needless activity to your primary patient mission? Are you doing what only you can do?

Questioning the status quo can be one of the most important aspects to growing your practice. If everything you currently do is sacred and immune to inspection or questioning, you're a prime candidate for burnout and early retirement. Practice is a process, not a destination. If you think you'll ever find the perfect procedure, the ultimate admitting form, or the flawless front desk person, dream on. First, they don't exist, and second, it's professional suicide. Once you become fixated, you start decaying like a spinal joint. Life is measured by motion, the ability to adapt and change, and a responsiveness that precludes mechanistic solutions and dogmatic "this-is-the-way-it's-done" attitudes–whether they come from me or anyone else. Lighten up and enjoy the ride. Getting there (since "there" doesn't exist) is the fun part. ■

THE MAN IN THE MOON

If it wasn't for the moon, we probably wouldn't have a space program. If all we saw when we looked to the heavens were the faraway stars, the effort to explore space probably wouldn't have been pursued. The moon was far enough to stimulate the imagination, yet close enough to be attainable. Setting reasonable goals that push our limits, but are achievable, can serve to motivate and inspire. Goals that are too easy or too ambitious don't fully harness our energy or creativity.

This notion of "reachability" is also important when giving chiropractic care recommendations. Without milestones, and a sense of measurable progress, many patients give up or remain uninspired to pursue a doctor's lofty recommendations completely enough to truly benefit from optimum health.

The goal setting process and establishing appropriate expectations of the recommended care program is usually provided during the patient's report of findings. Patients, accustomed to overnight results from ingesting medicine, need to have their expectations modified lest they think chiropractic doesn't work if instant results aren't achieved. Providing achievable goals, giving patients ways of measuring their progress, and assigning responsibilities, are key ingredients for giving effective instructions—which is essentially the purpose of a report of findings.

Richard Wurman, following up *Information Anxiety* has written, *Follow the Yellow Brick Road* which he details the five important considerations when giving instructions: Giver, Taker, Content, Channel, and Context.

Giver: Doctors presenting a report of findings must have a clear objective in mind for the outcome they want from this crucial patient interaction. Doctors overly concerned about whether they will be liked, or fearful that their recommendations won't be accepted, enter into the report with a strike against them. Similarly, doctors who begin their report suspecting that their recommendations have little chance of being acted upon by the patient, may end up sabotaging the communication, creating a self-fulfilling prophecy.

Often these and other doctor attitudes that impair the maximum impact of their report are the result of "owning" the patient's problem. When a new patient has headaches, many doctors incorrectly assume that by accepting the case, the patient's problem is now *their* problem. And while every effort should be made to convey compassion and a willingness to help, care must be taken so that the patient knows he or she has responsibilities too. Health restoration is as much or more the responsibility of the patient than the doctor. Purposely or inadvertently assuming too much responsibility for the patient's recovery dramatically affects the effectiveness of the report.

Taker: In our application of "giving directions" the taker is the patient. They are at the receiving end of the instructions affecting compliance in a report of findings setting. Ironically, many "givers" have difficulty empathizing with the patient sufficiently enough to achieve the rapport necessary for optimum communication. Many doctors easily forget the personality-distorting effects of pain and discomfort, or the judgment-hindering effect of feeling powerless; or the fear-producing effect of anticipating the diagnosis; or the worry-producing effect of the cost of their care; or the guilt-producing effect of spending so much money on themselves. The point is, few patients standing in front of your X-ray view box have their normal faculties. That college educated, middle manager with the low back problem may "look" like he is in full control, but he probably isn't.

This doesn't mean that you should reduce your "instructions" to baby talk. It just means that a large percentage of what you say either isn't being heard, properly interpreted, or remembered. The fact that most reports are primarily oral recitations is one of the biggest flaws of the one-time-report-of-findings approach to patient education!

Content: This is what has been the primary focus of management firms; what is *said* during the report. Sadly, many doctors "learn" a report and with the exception of the patient's name and particular health complaint, deliver pretty much the same report to every patient. Not only is this a lazy way of communicating to patients, eventually the report is delivered without the appropriate body language, passion, and conviction so critical to encoding the confidence and trust necessary for acceptance.

This fixation on scripted words isn't irrelevant, it's just superficial. I wonder how many times I've heard the story of the crusty old veteran doctor showing the same set of X-rays to every patient, growling, "You've got a bone out of place here and here. Now lie down and let's get started!" This may have worked for a previous generation of patients who cowered at the directives of anyone with a college degree, but not today.

Today, the foundation of any effective report of findings must be the answering of four basic patient questions: What's wrong with me? Can chiropractic help? If so, how long will it take? How much will it cost? The mistake many doctors make is avoiding the financial issues of chiropractic care. Ignoring this matter, or divorcing it from the care recommendations, is a cruel joke played out in countless offices by doctors embarrassed by what they charge their patients, or afraid the patient won't comply because of the financial policy. Not that money should be the focus of patient compliance, but it shouldn't be overlooked. It certainly isn't by patients!

Channel: This refers to the medium used to transmit the instructions. In that most report of findings are largely oral presentations complimented by an occasional X-ray with obscure pencil lines and angle measurements, they overlook the best channels for making an impact. Many doctors seem oblivious to the existence of fast-cutting

TV commercials, the emergence of MTV, and a decline in literacy. They are still relying on the narrow channel of an oral presentation or brochures containing an uninviting sea of gray type. Perhaps this channel is still effective for the generation that grew up in the "theater of the mind" days of radio, but today most patients want information fast, easy, and personally relevant. Newspaper readership is down just about everywhere, and virtually every month we hear the emergence of still another cable channel. The newspapers that *are* doing well, such as *USA Today* are full of captioned pictures and color graphics. They're not the newspapers our parents grew up with!

This suggests that video (or eventually CD-ROM) has a place in your report of findings communication efforts. If you're just going to have a "talking head," scrolling text, or meaningless special effects, don't bother. Not only has television made the public lazy, it's made them critical of amateur, home made presentations. A fifteen second clip on *America's Funniest Home Videos* might be interesting, but a stiff, ten minute talking head of the doctor behind his or her desk is deadly.

While technology will probably never replace the personalization and human connection of some type of oral presentation, consider adding media that can give your message more impact. Because the channel that is the richest and most memorable is visual, making your report more stimulating to the patient's eyes is your best bet at making your observations and recommendations understandable, memorable, and more likely to be acted upon.

Context: The fifth component of effective directions is to be sensitive to the context of the message. The challenge here is that most doctors have difficultly seeing their recommendations from the perspective of the patient. It's so easy (and wrong) to explain that their problem will require "three times a week for the first three weeks, then two times a week for the next two weeks, and then..." For starters, you don't have the foggiest notion how the patient will respond, how quickly the healing process will occur, or whether the patient will change other lifestyle aspects necessary for a speedy recovery. Secondly, in the context of a patient's life, the recommendations you make have a financial ramification that is often overlooked by doctors who receive their care without any impact to their monthly budget. Recognizing that patients aren't *living* to get adjusted is a major shift for most doctors!

The most effective communicators help translate abstract findings and recommendations into concepts that are relevant to the patient. Here, the use of metaphors and analogies that relate to the patient's occupation, hobbies, or key values is critical. Effective communicators use word pictures, models, and visual aids to help patients see their chiropractic care in personal terms.

Giving directions to patients is not unlike the ability to give directions and delegate responsibilities to staff members. Come to think of it, doctors who have good patient compliance, also seem to have staff members who rally along side the doctor and almost instinctively know what to do. But it's not instinct. It's the doctor's ability to give clear directions based on outcome.

Whether you're giving patients directions to your office, or your recommendations for care, offering landmarks and ways of assuring patients they're on the right course is important. "If you pass a large shopping mall, you've gone too far." Offer your care recommendations in bite-sized pieces with a clearly defined (and measurable) goal in mind. "At the next progressive examination in four weeks, I want to see this improve by at least ten degrees..."

The notion of having to continually earn the right to render care to a patient is a new idea for a whole generation of chiropractors. The days of making sweeping recommendations at your report of findings spanning months and months of care (conveniently paid for by a third party) are gone for good. Sure, give them the big picture and let them know that some type of lifetime care may be necessary, but give them smaller, achievable goals that they can support both intellectually and financially. Otherwise, not only are you kidding yourself, you're over-estimating your patients' resources and the value they place on their health. ■

THE TWELFTH VISIT

Offices interested in creating long term "client" relationships with their patients, have learned how to effectively manage the patient's twelfth visit in the office. If this crucial visit isn't handled properly, patient compliance suffers and the benefits of a chiropractic lifestyle are rarely enjoyed by patients.

For some offices it might be the tenth visit or the fifteenth visit. Pick a visit number at which a majority of your patients typically show progress, but are clearly not through with their care. At about this same point most patients are asking themselves, "How much longer am I going to need chiropractic care?" Since few patients will actually confront the doctor with this question, it is important to anticipate it and be prepared to deal with it. Waiting, thinking patients will obediently continue with rehabilitative care, and eagerly submit to maintenance care because you told them to do so at your report of findings, is naive.

Obviously, patient education is a critical ingredient in these proceedings. If patients don't understand the full nature and severity of their problem and the value of continuing care after symptomatic relief, they won't. Patients need to understand the underlying muscle damage that predisposes them to a relapse. Patients need to know about the length of time it takes to heal the soft tissues because these tissues have a poor blood supply. Patients need to appreciate the calcium salt deposition and bone remodeling that occurs from long standing spinal problems. Without this knowledge, patients can do nothing but trust how they *feel*, as a way to judge the necessity of continuing their care. Without this understanding, when the inevitable relapse occurs, patients naturally blame the doctor, chiropractic, or both.

Besides a systematic patient education effort on every visit, on or about the twelfth visit there should be a way patients can record their subjective assessment of their progress. There should be a re-examination emphasizing the positive findings from the initial examination. And finally a complete report to the patient with a revised treatment plan. Whether this is done on one visit, or spread between two seems less important than doing *something* to offer feedback to the patient. If the doctor ignores this type of accountability or overlooks the necessity of reaffirming the patient's commitment, don't expect the patient to continue with nonsymptomatic wellness care! With the focus over the last ten years on new patient acquisition, most seminars and management programs have overlooked this critical aspect of "keeping" patients.

A twelfth visit protocol is easy to create. The key is to pick a particular visit number to perform these functions and not to wait for a comment or specific patient action to prompt the procedures. I like the twelfth visit because it usually represents about one month's worth of care, patients are usually showing progress by then, and they are devising ways to disengage from the office. Here are some observations to keep in mind regardless of the visit number you choose:

Patient self-assessment: Create a simple one page form that patients can complete on the day of your progressive examination. Ask some questions that simply require checking boxes to indicate subjective aspects of their lives that have improved since beginning care. Find out if walking, sitting, standing, sleeping, driving, and other functions have improved. Have them check boxes indicating whether digestion, breathing, thinking, and other physiological functions have improved. Then have them rate their perception of their overall progress on a continuum from 0 (no improvement) to 10 (total recovery). Use this same form to uncover concerns, frustrations, or unanswered questions. Find out if they've tried to refer others. Ask what the office can do to make it easier for them to tell their friends about chiropractic. Finally, have the patient sign and date the form.

There are several reasons why you want a written record of the patient's subjective assessment of their condition. The first is getting patients to think about their progress. With the painful presenting symptoms largely gone, it's easy for many patients to overlook crediting chiropractic for their improvement! Another reason is to uncover potential topics that may need to be stressed in future adjusting room conversations. From a legal standpoint, having your patients assessment of their progress to date may be helpful in certain personal injury cases or disputes with patients who later claim their care wasn't helpful.

What if they overrate their progress? That's the other aspect of continuing patient education. Your patient education responsibilities don't end at the completion of your second visit report of findings! If you want long term compliance, you must continue to explain the process and time needed to effect muscle and soft tissue healing.

Re-examination: Use much the same protocol you employ for your initial new patient admitting examination. The focus now is on those tests with initial positive findings and other objective orthopedic, neurological, and chiropractic tests. As you perform each examination, remind the patient what you're measuring, and why.

This re-examination is very important for more reasons than the obvious. When there is injury or noticeable restricted motion, many patients naturally curb their activities. As patients receive care, this self-policed moderation can fool them into thinking their recovery is happening faster than it actually is. Pain relief can be relatively quick when normal flexion and extension are unconsciously avoided. Because many tests evaluate the full limits of motion or sensitivity, when discomfort is encountered during the examination process patients realize more healing is necessary.

The purpose of the progress examination isn't to hurt the patient! Besides gathering information for comparative results, the examination process helps patients more accurately "feel" the extent of their recovery so far.

A frequent question I get at seminars is about performing a post X-ray examination. And while the profession is replete with dogma on this topic and many doctors justify not X-raying the patient so as to avoid "needless" radiation, many patients appreciate some type of progress X-ray examination. Are structural improvements possible in twelve visits? Often. Are functional improvements possible on flexion/extension views? Should be. Offices with large numbers of wellness patients often take post films at some point along the way because they are confident their technique works. Ask some patients if they're interested. Risk finding out the truth!

Progress Report: Like your initial report of findings, some form of patient education is helpful prior to your report so you can avoid repetitious explanations. There are many video programs available to accomplish this for you. And like your initial report of findings, the purpose of the report is to review and compare your (S)ubjective and (O)bjective examination findings, (A)ssess their progress, and offer a (P)lan for continued care.

When reviewing your patients subjective evaluation of their progress, compare their admitting paperwork complaints with the form you asked them to complete prior to your re-examination. While it may be only three or four weeks, most patients quickly forget what they were feeling on their first visit or two. Remind them, congratu-lating them on their progress, and of course give chiropractic and their inborn healing ability the credit.

Next, review your pre- and post-objective findings. Because the results are easily quantifiable, orthopedic test results can be very effective when communicating with patients. Compare three things. Compare your initial findings with your most recent findings with the measurements normally considered average. The point here is to acknowledge their progress, while reminding them that additional care may be needed to reach total recovery. Without this information, patients have no way of justifying continued care if they are free from pain.

When making and sharing your assessment, the third component of your progress report, it is important to acknowledge any apparent progress, offer hope if you are inclined to think further care will produce measurable improvement, and either concur with or dispute the patient's own evaluation of their recovery.

Because most patients are rarely in tip-top condition before suffering the injury or health complaint, it may be important to distinguish between how nearly they've reached pre-accident status and how close they are to optimum function.

The last part of your report is offering your plan for continued care. There are only a few choices. Will continued care require the same, greater, or lesser visit frequency? If so, justify your conclusion with your patients so they understand and agree. Make your recommendations in the same bite-sized increments of ten or twelve visits, so there are clear milestones along the way, accompanied by some type of repeated objective measurement of their progress.

If a patient isn't showing the progress you'd normally expect, you have the obligation to either refer to some other specialist or to another chiropractor who uses a different technique. The patient's needs come before your ego or professional esteem. Just remember, a patient or two who don't respond isn't an indictment or even a sign of failure. Choosing *not* to refer out is a sign of failure!

Progress examination reports help improve compliance and provide welcomed milestones for patients to judge their recovery. Without a clearly defined procedure, patients are more likely to drop out, resulting in an apparent need for confrontational recall procedures. By then it's too late. After all, how many cash-paying maintenance care patients have your past recall procedures generated? ∎

FOUR PATIENT
EDUCATION FALLACIES

It doesn't take long before every practitioner learns the importance of patient education. It's easy for doctors in practice for five years or more to forget the long term benefits of a consistent patient education program. Those offices with roller coaster statistics are often guilty of doing what they know works (patient education) only when they "need" to do it.

On an especially memorable episode of *The Cosby Show*, Dr. Huxtable was explaining how wasteful this starting and stopping approach can be. Apparently, Theo had decided to wait until right before his exams to begin studying. It seems that no amount of convincing could change Theo's behavior until Dad used a metaphor. He likened this short-term thinking to the enormous amounts of fuel that jet aircraft consume during take off (cramming before the test). Once the jet reaches cruising altitude it takes much less energy (daily studying). Similarly, a consistent system of patient education requires a minimum amount of energy and frees the doctor and staff to concentrate on the more important aspects of patient care. Without effective patient education, the doctor, staff, and financial resources are consumed by a constant focus on new patient acquisition rituals.

Yet, for many doctors, patient education sounds like work. Which is probably why so few invest in patient education. If you don't have a consistent, systematized way of doing it, then it probably *is* too much work. Is discipline required? Of course. Are their disappointments? Naturally. Do your words occasionally fall on deaf ears? Sure. Yet, if you take your responsibility as a teacher seriously, you have a professional obligation to educate your patients. The media won't. The state and national associations don't seem to. You're it.

There are several fallacies about patient education that need to be identified, lest you misunderstand what I mean by patient education.

The *I-told-them-once* fallacy. This is the mistaken notion that once you tell patients about subluxations and show them their X-rays, your patient education responsibilities are over. Few patients will appreciate the spine and its role in health as much as you after a single exposure to an oral presentation! If your patient education efforts are limited to the first couple of visits while patients are still somewhat apprehensive, suspicious, or distracted by their symptoms, don't expect them to retain the material! While it may be old fashioned, the "tell 'em what you're going to tell 'em, tell 'em, and then tell 'em what you told 'em" is an adage that still rings true. Create a plan to talk about some aspect of chiropractic on every visit.

The *I-showed-them-a-video* fallacy. Here, the doctor has introduced some technology to make the presentation of chiropractic more consistent, and if properly designed, give it more impact. If the video isn't merely a "talking head" it has the potential of making the message more understandable and memorable. Yet, without continual follow up and relating the information in the video to the patient's condition on subsequent visits, the use of video can seem out of place or appear like a sales session. While video can help avoid repetitious explanations so the doctor can concentrate on other aspects of patient care, video must reflect the philosophy and practice approach of the doctor. It is not a panacea and will never replace other types of "low-tech" patient communications.

The *I-have-posters-and-pamphlets-everywhere* fallacy. When doctors litter their offices with chiropractic tracts and brochures, and fill every available wall space with posters, they may assume that patients will learn chiropractic principles simply by osmosis. This patient-education-by-proximity approach is ineffective too. While it's true that the walls (ceilings?) of your office should be used to communicate your unique vision and approach to health, these tools must be referred to regularly or patients tune them out. Posters must be referred to. Brochures must be presented. Spinal models must be touched. Like a shovel that doesn't move dirt until it is used properly, patient education tools don't move patients to make better decisions about their health until they are used properly. Because these efforts are rarely rewarded with immediate results, our penchant for instant gratification is not affirmed. If your sense of time is no broader than the two or three weeks it takes to effect symptomatic improvement, you'll never harvest the bounty that relentless patient education can offer.

The "They-don't-care" fallacy. This is the notion that patients don't seem interested in anything more than pain relief, so educating patients is a waste of time. When doctors reflect this school of thought they have actually given up on themselves, not their patients. Think back to one of the worse teachers in school. Students can tell when the teacher isn't having fun or has neglected to update his or her notes. Worse, if the teacher doesn't take the effort to make the information relevant, then students (patients) react in a predictable manner. Are you making your patient education efforts germane to your patients' lives?

These four patient education fallacies can be found throughout the profession–among new doctors and experienced veterans. Patient education is one of the critical elements of a successful practice, especially today, as more and more patients are having to finance their care out of their own pockets. What's incredible is that effective patient communications is such a small part (or totally absent) from the curricula of today's chiropractic colleges. This critical missing link will continue to sabotage more and more new doctors in today's increasingly competitive marketplace.

Clearly, the best patient communicators have the best practices. Why not model those who depend upon optimum customer "education" for their livelihood? Ask any advertising agency or marketing director how to help patients "get it" and they will reveal two key approaches: impact or repetition, or a combination of both.

Impact: When the car company bungy jumps an automobile off a bridge, it's an attempt to give their message impact. When Pepsi, Kodak, Sprint or other companies use celebrities, it's to give their message impact. There are many ways giving your chiropractic message impact through the use of strong visuals, drama, humor, timing, volume, and others. Waving your hands in front of the X-ray view box isn't enough.

Repetition: Everyone who has watched television for any length of time knows about this approach. Repeating a consistent message for a long enough period of time and people will know how to "spell relief" or "who deserves a break today." Unfortunately for many patients, the only patient education they receive is a one-time oral presentation at the report of findings. No wonder they drop out of care once their symptoms improve!

Obviously the best patient education strategy is to combine both impact and repetition. For many it means rethinking the report of findings and giving it more impact than genuflecting in front of the X-ray view box. It will mean saying something on every visit to make the patient's biomechanical problem relevant to their lifestyles. It will mean questioning the status quo and abandoning the path of least resistance. For most it will mean taking their role as teachers more seriously. ■

GETTING THROUGH
TO PATIENTS

Virtually every doctor who recognizes the importance of patient education has been frustrated by their attempts to help patients "get" the chiropractic message. It seems that anything short of a Vulcan Mind Meld is ineffective or so short lived as to be meaningless. Certainly those doctors who have given up on patient education, taking the path of least resistance of pain relief and immediate dismissal, have grappled with this challenge. Ironically, what new doctors learn upon graduation as they begin their real education at the School of Hard Knocks, is that getting patients well is the easy part. Communicating with and motivating patients is the hard part, something barely addressed in chiropractic colleges obsessed with merely equipping students to pass state board examinations.

What apparently all too many forget is that attached to those thirty-one pairs of nerves that exit the spine is a cerebral cortex. This volitional animal, with its medical training since birth and real world concerns of time and money, controls compliance based on considerations other than biomechanics, better posture, or even preventing the degeneration of spinal neglect. One of the most important choices doctors make is whether to cave into this reality or fight it.

In the glory days of easy insurance money, too many chiropractors succumbed to the expediency and profitability of running a pain relief clinic. With countless more $100 deductible patients waiting in the wings, patient education was seen as a luxury or a waste of time. "Patient's don't want to know about chiropractic, they just want out of pain," they reasoned. Poor attendance at spinal care classes, and complaints about documentary-length videos were further proof that patient education was an unnecessary distraction. Instead, hopes for the future were put on the outcome of the suit against the American Medical Association, inserts in *Reader's Digest*, increasingly larger yellow page ads, and sophisticated insurance billing software. And so, almost a generation later, chiropractic is still perceived as a second rate, unscientific, alternative, last-resort form of pain relief. A valuable opportunity was squandered by a profession of Lone Rangers, many who reasoned they could *buy* acceptance by sporting Rolex watches and driving expensive cars, like *real* doctors.

Today, many are learning the hard way what chiropractors before insurance equality knew: patient education is the key to a growing practice. Those without a strong philosophical background, or introverts with poor communication skills are finding this new environment especially challenging. Fortunately, communication skills can be learned. And those who have already mastered effective patient communications, regularly use impact, repetition, and passion to help patients understand chiropractic.

The Power of Impact

When Nikita Khrushchev pounded his shoe on the podium at the United Nations, he gave his message impact. Here are some less drastic ways the best chiropractic communicators give their message maximum impact:

Drama: Stories are some of the most powerful ways to communicate values and ideas. Fairy tales, parables, allegories, and even television sitcoms offer a forum to explain or present a point of view with powerful mnemonics. This is why testimonials can be so effective.

Exaggeration: "You're too sick to come to the office! Oh no!" exaggerates the front desk assistant. "You're planning to miss your next appointment!?! What do you suppose that's going to do to your recovery?" asks the doctor with an expression of mock horror. Here, the motive is to take some casual comment or observation and exaggerate the reaction. Make little things seem huge and big concerns small.

Use pictures: Television, magazines, and our popular culture have created a generation of visually-oriented patients. An oral report doesn't offer the same punch of well chosen visuals. Use metaphorical representations of the pathologies that occur with aberrant spinal biomechanics and watch patient understanding improve. Get beyond the obvious "bone out of place" model communicated by X-rays.

Humor: Laughter may be the best medicine, but it's also a great catalyst for learning. While there is nothing humorous about a herniated disc or a bone spur, use humor when you can. No one said you can't laugh while you're saving the world!

Involvement: This is the easiest, yet most over-looked way to give your message impact. Have each patient "phase-place" their spine, telling you the phase of degeneration it's in, based on your videos or posters. Have patients write your recommendations for care in their own handwriting on your report handout. In many subtle ways you can increase a patient's compliance by involving them more directly in their care.

Volume: Related to drama, use the loudness of your voice as a way to communicate the seriousness of your recommendations. Sometimes a whisper can have more impact than a shout.

Five senses: We learn through the five senses. The more you can involve the patient's other senses, besides the way they "feel," the more you can increase the impact of your recommenda tions. Are you using taste and smell in your office? Have patients touch a bone spur on a spinal model. Brainstorm other ways with your staff.

Pattern interrupt: One way to draw attention to your message and give it more impact is to create what psychologists call a pattern interrupt. Moving your educational wall posters to a new location each week is a pattern interrupt. Drawing attention to your referral board each week by posting the names of famous personalities is a pattern interrupt. Keep the office changing and alive.

The Cumulative Effects of Repetition

Another way the most effective communicators get their message across is to constantly repeat it. Television advertisers understand this axiom completely. Because of repetition, we all know how to spell relief (R-O-L-A-I-D-S), and that Dominos Delivers, and that "Nothing beats a great pair of Leggs," and countless other slogans that clog our brain.

More than simply saying the same thing over and over again, effective communicators use a variety of techniques to benefit from the cumulative effects of repetition:

Tell 'em what you're going to tell 'em. While some doctors shy away from this basic communication axiom, using the examination process as a way of foreshadowing the contents of your report of findings can improve patient acceptance. Too many doctors reason that revealing the examination results without the context of a complete report gives away the "punch line." Not true. Since chiropractic is something new for most patients, you'll find patients more willing to participate if you avoid numbing them with too much information at the report, and instead, show more of your "cards" during the examination process.

Use a variety of media. Here the repetition idea is to make sure that wherever the patient turns, a consistent message is communicated. Advertisers use this approach by using the same type of music on radio and television, the same type of graphics in their television commercials, on billboards, and product packaging, etc. The use of repetition in this "campaign approach" makes the product or service more accepted because it is seen in so many places.

Harnessing Your Passion

A key ingredient of all communication approaches is to insure that the message communicated on a verbal level matches the message communicated on a non-verbal level. This need for congruency is often why procedures and scripts taught at seminars don't work for some practitioners. If doctors or staff members do not "own" the script, the philosophy behind it, or cannot match the appropriate physical manifestations that should accompany key phrases, then the patient senses discord and the message is perceived as unbelievable.

If you study the best communicators (Anthony Robbins, Martin

Luther King, Ross Perot, Rush Limbaugh, etc.) you can tell that their convictions run to the depths of every sinew. Because of this congruency, it gives their messages incredible impact. If you're not fired up about chiropractic, doubt the value of wellness care, are afraid to take post X-rays, or are holding back in any other way, patients can "smell" it. Besides sabotaging the moment, your thinly disguised lack of commitment becomes a self-fulfilling prophecy, as patients seem distant, drop out, don't refer, or just disappear without explanation. In the same way animals can tell when you're afraid or simply not grounded, so can patients. ■

IN PURSUIT OF PASSION

It seems so odd to have to mention it, but what patients really want is passion. They want to see the visible evidence of your commitment to chiropractic. They want to see their doctor totally committed to his or her profession. A doctor going through the motions, a slave to the overhead, or someone who doesn't seem to be having fun is less than inspirational. Besides sabotaging compliance, a lack of passion interferes with the healing process.

Patients are rarely more excited about chiropractic than their doctor.

At seminars I hear, "Gee Bill, you seem so passionate and committed to what you're doing. Where do you get all your energy and excitement?" they ask, as if I've found a place at the mall that sells passion!

"Why were you placed on this planet?" I answer.

That's right. If you don't know why you're here, it's hard to align yourself with the fundamental forces in control of the universe. It is having access to this energy that facilitates daily activity and makes it fulfilling. Otherwise you're simply swimming upstream against the current.

Nothing beautiful is ever forced.

Tapping into this source is one of the most important spiritual journeys any of us take. It's rarely accomplished in hotel ballrooms with hundreds of other participants, walking on a bed of hot coals, or whatever is the latest seminar gimmick. It requires honesty, discipline, and the ability to confront your greatest fears. It is a critical rite of passage. Only when you risk this introspection and inventory of talent can you generate the passion necessary for the success and the fulfillment you deserve.

How do you know when you've uncovered your purpose? Your mission?

When there is a sense of effortless accomplishment. When you are in flow. When your level of service to others exceeds your own rewards. When you love what you do so much, you'd do it without compensation. When your motives are pure. When you seem connected to patients and you're less worried about the financial aspects of a case than the welfare of the patient. When you finally can think big enough that you're not worried about what others think. When energy is leveraged so powerfully that projects and situations seem self-propelled by their own need to *be*.

This is when practice is fun.

Here are some suggestions to get the passion back in your life. Ways to recover the sense of purpose and idealism you had back in school. Suggestions to begin having a life:

Not a dress rehearsal: First you must recognize the urgency of the situation. This is your life we're talking about here. Suffering and bondage is not part of God's plan. In no other part of nature do we see these confining attitudes. Freedom, growth, and unabandoned life is all around us. The *Proverbs* writer who observed "Without vision the people perish" is quoted often and its truth is ageless. If you're not having fun you're letting a part of yourself die. Do something! If you're waiting until... or, you're going to let that staff member go who's sabotaging patient compliance if... or, you're going to start working out when... you're simply lying to yourself. Do it now. Clean house. Draw the line. Get on with it. Procrastinating is a form of lying to oneself that drains you of energy and distracts your focus.

Review your past: In Arthur Miller's book, *The Truth About You*, he tackles this important issue. He suggests the first place to start in your search for purpose is to review your life. Create a list of situations in each decade of your life (ages 1-10, 10-20, etc.), in which

166

you felt "connected" and fulfilled. During this brainstorming stage simply record events that gave you "goose bumps" or a sense of purpose. Was it learning a new skill, testing a limit, exceeding someone's expectations, or building something? Did these situations involve people, things, or places? List as many of these occasions as you can for each decade of your life. Then evaluate the list. Any common denominators through the years? If you can't find a pattern, show your list to someone else. Then, simply make sure these revelations are woven into your life. If serving others in your chiropractic career can't accommodate it (highly unlikely), move on! Don't allow the investment made in your professional schooling to limit you. If you're not fired up about chiropractic, chiropractic will get along quite nicely without you. Spread your wings. Become all you can be.

Enlarge your vision: Think big! Today you'd be surprised how many doctors neglect to even include their telephone area codes on their business cards! A big vision can galvanize those around you to contribute more. People like being part of something big. Little visions are for little people. If you're idea of success is to be able to pay the bills, it's likely you'll be sentenced to nothing but. The more you ask of yourself the more you become. Set higher standards. Welcome the uncomfortable feeling of thinking big. Nothing great was ever accomplished by worrying about what the neighbors think or always being right. Stop thinking about yourself. If you're depressed, it's because you're probably thinking about yourself instead of serving others.

Confront your greatest fear: Limiting most of us is fear. Sometimes we are aware of its hold on us. Other times it is submerged below the conscious level and we only occasionally bump up against it. Everyone has some type of fear. Even those who appear fearless tread ahead anyway, bringing their fears with them. The differenc is that they don't allow False Evidence Appearing Real to stop the Interestingly, when you confront your fear of public speaking, taJ post X-rays, calling patients after their first adjustment, adju children, or who knows what else, the fear disappears. That's how you acquire the self-confidence to project the excitement that patients want. The world clears a wide path for those who are fearless. The world is hungry for leadership.

Know what you want: It never ceases to amaze me how many doctors begin a relationship, set a policy, or enter into a situation without a clear outcome in mind. What do you want? And listing what you *don't* want won't work. The world works in positives. Get a piece of paper and write it down. Something clicks in the brain when you articulate your objective on a piece of paper. It becomes real. The number of people who don't regularly set goals is criminal. The aimlessness and susceptibility to opportunity chasing (water purifiers, rehab centers, vitamins, pillows, etc.) is greatest among those most unsure of what they really want. Those who know their purpose, invent their future by scripting it through the goal setting process.

Reframe your situation: One doctor I know was having difficulty regaining his passion for practice after 12 years of successfully shepherding a sizable number of patients through his personal injury business. As he watched his practice slowly erode he felt impotent to identify the barrier preventing the excitement he wanted. "As you convert your practice from insurance to a cash/family orientation, think of it as starting over–like creating a new practice from the ground up," I suggested. For the first time that morning a smile crossed his face. Since then he hasn't looked back. New patient problems can be seen as patient retention problems. Cancellations are opportunities. Staff members quitting is a chance to find someone better. Discontinue "half empty" thinking and replace it with "half full" thinking.

Increase your physical capacity: It's impossible to project a high level of excitement and commitment if you're running out of steam at 3:00 PM. Being in tip-top physical condition is just as important as having the proper "head space." Lose those extra pounds and improve your ability to exude the vitality and confidence patients want to see in their doctor. Become a living testimonial to the value of a chiropractic lifestyle. Walk 30% faster.

Communicate your vision: This is an overlooked aspect of the leadership responsibilities you automatically assume by being a doctor. Just about everyone you encounter is prepared to contribute their energies in pursuit of a worthy goal. Sharing your vision for the future of your practice and setting specific attainable goals, serves as a powerful rallying point for others in your sphere of influence. Simply put, your staff and patients can't help you attain what you want unless they know what you want! Want more cash-paying wellness patients? Let the world know. Want more pediatric patients? Make sure all your patients know. Want more ideal patients? Make sure your staff knows what your idea of an ideal patient is!

We shouldn't have to become dependent on a steady diet of "motivational" seminars to remain excited about life. If you can't see the miracles around you, you're not looking hard enough. The most successful practices are those that are fueled by a passionate doctor. It is something you cannot buy, lease, or rent. That's why it inspires patients so effectively. It is the language of unbridled love and service. ■

DISCRETIONARY ENERGY

In Hal Rosenthal's book, *The Customer Comes Second*, he observes that all the recent focus on the customer (patient) service has been misdirected. He suggests that employees come first. Employees treat customers (patients) the way their supervisors (doctors) treat them. If the boss is authoritarian and untrusting, staff members use the same level of hostility towards customers. Yet, he intones, the reverse is true too. At its most fundamental, it is a question of leadership. Poor leadership creates inattentive, unresponsive, and detached employees. Great leadership fosters committed, enthusiastic, and conscientious career-oriented employees. The hallmark of offices with low staff turnover and delighted patients who refer is the way doctors tap into the "discretionary energy" of their staff.

Your car mechanic takes the effort to show you how proper tire inflation will improve your gas mileage. Your wait person gently steers you away from a menu item that she knows is poorly prepared. Your hotel clerk asks you whether you'd prefer a room with a view of the gorgeous sunsets or the beautiful sunrises. These are examples of discretionary energy. They require the front line service provider to go beyond the required and expected. When ordinary or expected levels of service are rendered, the event is barely noticed by the customer. When extraordinary service (requiring discretionary energy) is delivered, it is memorable and provides customers with the motive to remain loyal and refer others. Getting staff members (and doctors!) to embrace this servant attitude and regularly deploy their discretionary energy seems elusive. It is not something that can be ordered or mandated by office policy. It cannot be obtained by threats or keeping staff members uninformed about what's going on. It is earned.

In a chiropractic setting, discretionary energy prompts staff members to remember little details or preferences of each patient and make their visit more pleasant. It's when the doctor takes the time to call the patient after the first adjustment. It's when a staff member bends the rules just a little to help solve a patient's problem. It's when staff members step in to help a patient's temporary transportation problem. It's the ability to recognize the thousands of little opportunities that reveal themselves when you're working with other people. It can't be ordered or policed. Each staff member decides if their additional energy reserves will be used in the service of patients, or taken home to a hobby, the bowling alley, or squandered in front of the a set.

Many chiropractic management firms seem to overlook ways of empowering doctors to harness this important type of energy in their staffs. Whether they'd rather more directly serve the needs of the doctor who pays them, incorrectly assume creating long term staff relationships is impossible, or that they don't know how to adapt to this management reality, is difficult to know. In the past, quickly training low-wage women to process patients and paperwork was the only goal. Staff members rarely stayed more than a year. Burnout was epidemic. Today, one thing is clear. As insurance continues to be less of a factor and chiropractic enters the free enterprise market economy, it will be those offices able to cultivate the discretionary energy of their staff that will enjoy a competitive edge.

Here are some ideas that can help prepare the soil so discretionary energy can grow and prosper in a chiropractic environment:

Spirit: This has to do with shared values. It is essential that doctors and staff share a similar value system if the most frequently mentioned patient complaint about staff members is to be avoided: turnover. You've seen it a million times. The potential new staff member has incredible skills. He or she can alphabetize better than a dictionary. Or he or she has a winsome way with delinquent patients.

The only problem is they have a foul mouth, worship trees, or think piercing any body part for a decorative "earring" is, well, attractive. Too bad. The foundation of long term doctor/staff relationships (and long term doctor/patient relationships) is a shared value system.

Belonging to a team: Many suggest that belonging to a group is a fundamental yearning for most of us. If you want to tap into the discretionary energy of your staff, help them to assimilate into your team. That's more difficult than it sounds. Think back to the Apollo mission to the moon. Consider the incredible teamwork required. Give people a big vision and watch their commitment increase. Small dreams (making a salary, getting by, paying the bills, etc.) attract small people. Big dreams attract big contributors and inspire the best in everyone.

Access to information: I continue to find it amazing how many staff members are kept in the dark regarding some of the most basic office information. You'd be surprised how many staff members are not under care themselves and haven't the foggiest idea what chiropractic is! Worse, the office mission statement and practice values are never articulated and even statistics are considered state secrets. Staff members see the big checks coming in the mail, but rarely see what it costs to run the office. When information isn't shared, staff members are left to their imagination—with counterproductive results. "Why knock myself out," wonder many staff members, "when I'm getting paid peanuts and the doctor is making a million dollars a year?"

Big vision: We all want to be part of something bigger than ourselves. This desire to belong and identify is a powerful force exploited by sports teams, religious cults, swat teams, political parties, and other groups. Yet, instead of taking opinion polls and worrying about what employees (and patients) think, everyone is looking to their doctor for direction and leadership. Leaders are much more interested in doing the right things, than doing things right. If you want to tap into the energy reserves of your staff, make sure everyone knows the target you're aiming for. Take a stand. State your position. Share a vision.

Safe risk taking: With a clearly articulated vision, staff members can be more confident and resourceful in making the millions of tiny judgment calls required. Each staff member should feel that it is safe to make mistakes in non-life or death situations. Staff members should be encouraged to try new ways of getting things done. Break the rules? Of course—when it's appropriate. Staff members need to know that when something goes wrong the "system" (or lack of one) is as much to blame as they are. Creative new solutions and a "can-do attitude" thrive in environments which encourage appropriate risk-taking. Staff members give 110% only when it's safe.

Appropriate acknowledgement: Funny, but staff members rarely give that "extra something special" unless someone notices it and acknowledges it. Fortunately for some staff members all it takes is to have a patient say, "I enjoy coming here just to see your bright smile." Yet, for most staff members it requires more than a chance comment from a particularly delighted patient. Again, this is the responsibility of the doctor. Aggressively search out occasions to thank, congratulate, and be delighted by things your staff says and does. Virtually every study conducted on employee motivation suggests that money is much less of a motivator then praise, encouragement, and working with appreciative people.

Doctors who whine that "all they really want to do is adjust" discover that their dream can come true, if they are willing to put into place office systems and employee training that can leverage their time and talent. It is hard for staff members to bring their discretionary energy to bear on the direction of the office if they have to handle everything three times: first when a problem is presented, second when it is described to the doctor, and finally a third time when they act on the doctor's direction. No wonder few staff members use their discretionary energy—it gets used up just trying to get through a typical day! ■

DEEP RUTS

Psychologists who study the success habits of the most visible business, sports, and entertainment leaders, talk of "the shadow." The shadow is a fringe area of our lives in which we hide our fears, our shortcomings as parents, lovers, and leaders of others. The shadow contains unaddressed issues that affect our personal, behind-the-scenes life. It is this shadow that grows as we devote increasing amounts of energy to our careers, at the expense of our families, our personal health, spiritual well-being, hobbies, and other seemingly "non-essential" aspects of our lives. This preoccupation, while effective at producing the visible signs and trappings of "success," sows the seeds for burnout and emptiness. Doctors who admit to the shadow recognize large amounts of energy are being used to cover up shortcomings as a boss, a husband or wife, or those deep dark secrets we think no one else has.

Knowing and recognizing the symptoms of imbalance between our professional and personal lives and doing something about it, is easier said than done. We all tend to stick with things that "work." Convincing the owner of a huge multi-clinic empire to change from the authoritarian, dictatorial management style that served him during the creation of his chiropractic kingdom, is likely to fall on deaf ears. (He's out of business now, still unwilling to admit his own role in the demise of his organization.) Changing and giving up attitudes, procedures, or policies that are no longer effective is very difficult. Like the office that got into the expensive habit of advertising for new patients, it is frightening to contemplate discontinuing. "Will I still get enough new patients?" "How long do I give it before I resume advertising if it doesn't work?" The doubts and fears are quite revealing–if we'll take the time to look. Instead, our temptation is to submerge these concerns into the shadow. "If it's not broken, why fix it" we reckon. And life goes on.

As leaders of patients and staff members, doctors have been coaxed into projecting a persona of total control, confidence, and unfailing perfection. While many new doctors find this role unsettling at first, it isn't long before they "buy into" this model and assume the expectations of those around them. Soon, after a string of "successes" with patients these notions of omniscience become more comfortable. Finally, they've stepped over an unseen boundary between the *facilitator* of health to the *grantor* of health. This is a heady and egotistically affirming position. With each passing month it becomes easier and easier to forget the words of Dr. Clay Thompson who said, "The doctor enters with the patient."

It's not just patients. Relationships with staff members soon fall under the spell of power and position. This is revealed by staff members who are afraid of the doctor or who are kept in a constant state of uncertainty about their job security. This creates an atmosphere of distrust that sabotages the synergistic $1 + 1 = 3$ possibilities of an office team. Again, changing or abandoning this unhealthy attitude or work habit can be very difficult. The very reason a doctor can so easily assume this position of power and influence, is the very reason they often don't recognize it even exists! Many advisors that surround you are afraid to volunteer the bad news for fear, like Saddam Hussein's messenger's of bad news, that they too will be metaphorically "shot" for telling the truth. Sadly, this little class warfare is being acted out in all too many offices. This "I'll-pretend-I'm-successful-and-everyone-around-me-will-too" covers up a major feedback loop of information and forces everyone to pretend the emperor is wearing a well tailored suit.

While there are few chiropractic colleges, management programs, or one-day seminars that address this fundamental issue, avoiding this trap of "success" can help grow the practice more effectively than superior adjusting skills, office location, or streamlined procedures. The doctor's comfort with him or herself and the willingness to confront this basic issue of personal "success" is a significant indicator of the health of the practice. Doctors in denial rarely "get it" until it's too late. "Why don't patient's refer?" "How come no one likes me?" "Why is it so hard to keep staff members?" "What am I doing wrong?"

The fact is, chiropractic is entering a market economy in which the forces of supply and demand, personality, energy level, passion, appearance, pricing, and other factors are going to play a larger role than ever before. To adapt and respond appropriately to these issues requires a doctor in touch with reality, who is grounded, centered, and open to new ideas. The aloof "doctorly" doctor of the past need not apply. Old style dictatorial management, communication, and interpersonal skills will not serve you in the future. The chilling fact is, what worked ten years ago is not likely to work in the future. The world has changed. Have you?

If you recognize you need to make some changes, here are some practical action steps to help you evolve into a doctor more likely to survive and thrive in the difficult-to-predict future ahead:

Admit mistakes. Lighten up a little. You're merely human. Even though you deal with the life and death forces of health, you are not perfect. When mistakes or oversights occur, admit them. Ironically, it enhances believability and respect from those around you. Instead of putting yourself on a pedestal, come down off your high horse to build rapport and mingle with the little people.

*"***I don't know.***"* Related to making mistakes, but not as drastic, is the ability to admit that you don't have an answer. Chiropractors, with their "cause" orientation are always quick to answer any question thrown at them by their patients. This "Mr. Know-it-all" attitude tends to separate you from those you serve in a way that is counterproductive. No wonder many people think chiropractors believe they can cure everything! We always have an answer or a quick come

back. It's all right to admit you don't know something. "I don't remember that from my second quarter pathology class, but I'll look it up and get back with you tomorrow."

Coach and mentor. Actions speak louder than words and like teenagers who only give you polite attention about your anti-drug stance while you're holding your scotch on the rocks, don't expect patients to believe you if you're carrying 20 pounds extra or still smoking. Patients are looking to you and your staff for guidance about what you believe and do. You must become someone that your patients and staff would like to become. Are you?

Sanction risk taking. The fear of failure haunts your staff and your patients. If you want innovation, creativity, and excitement to greet you when you enter your office in morning, make sure your staff and patients feel safe. Safety may be simply mentioning your appreciation. Or affirming your patients decisions to show up regularly for their appointments. Make sure that trying new ideas (and the potential for failure that always accompanies them) is recognized and nurtured. The real failure is in not trying.

Show appreciation. Another common sense idea is to remember to say "please" and "thank you." It may be because of my upbringing, but I'm inclined to say thank you to anyone who helps me in even the slightest way. The cabin attendants who served an unappreciated flight, the staff member who simply does what's expected, or the customer who points out a shortcoming in my seminar. "Thank you!" encourages more openness and reality checks. Be sure to show your appreciation. This is even more important as your success increases. All too often people are inclined to tell you what you *want* to hear, instead of what you *need* to hear. Make sure you reward those who are bold enough to tell the truth.

Be humble. It's tempting to get sucked up into the notion that you're the one responsible for the patient's recovery! Buying into this idea and becoming the lightening rod of their appreciation is alluring, but perhaps a big mistake. First, it draws attention to you instead of chiropractic, and second, it sets you up to accept an equal dose of disappointment on those occasions when chiropractic doesn't work. This is a double edged sword that few doctors recognize. Chiropractic is bigger than you. Make sure your patients know it.

Accept compliments. On the other side of the coin, be ready to acknowledge your role in the healing process. Remember how desperate patients felt when they consulted you on their first visit. Recognize the hope you have given them. Many doctors who reach the upper levels of "success" often have difficulty accepting a compliment. Honor the patient's observations and accept your role as facilitator. Balancing this with the notion of being humble takes conscious attention.

Meet your family. Your family is more important than all your patients combined. Without your family you lose an important touchstone with reality. There's nothing more disarming when I'm feeling just a notch above the rest of the world than to be reminded to clean out the cat box. This is the great equalizer. Make sure that you take enough time along the way to nurture and raise your family. Make sure your children know your name. Rarely do they care about the extra time and energy you give the practice to produce the money for the better cut of meat, the club membership, the nicer clothes, or the faster car. They want you. Not the stuff.

Strengthen your spiritual foundation. While most management programs and seminars successfully sidestep this issue, if your spiritual life is in a mess, your practice is too. Whether your strength comes from Christ or from some other power greater than you, acknowledge and nurture this aspect of your life. I happen to believe there are absolute rights and wrongs. Denying this and entering a world of relativity where "as long as it doesn't hurt anyone else it's okay with me," invites trouble.

Take a few moments to step aside and see where you are and where you're going. Like the sign posted at the beginning of a well-worn old jeep trail in the Colorado Rocky Mountains that says, "Pick your ruts carefully," it may be time to reevaluate the path you've chosen. Is it taking you where you want to go? ■

PATIENT GARDENING

Jesus tells the parable of the four soils in Matthew 13, 3-8. Some seeds fell on the path and were eaten by the birds. Other seeds landed on rocks and were unable to grow in the hot sun. Still other seeds settled among thorns and were crowded out by the weeds. And a few seeds fell on fertile soil and grew to return its harvest up to 100 fold. This agriculture based illustration made it easy to understand his message. It's a famous parable that describes how your chiropractic message sometimes falls on deaf ears and other times takes hold and inspires an entire family to begin and remain under care.

Bill Moyers, in his book *Healing And The Mind* and its companion PBS television series, was quite taken by the Eastern notion of viewing the body and its health, as a garden. A garden to be cultivated and nurtured. It's a wonderful metaphor that can be applied to cultivating the health of one's practice too. First you have to decide what you want to grow! The vegetable seed packets you buy at the gardening store are commonly sold by vegetable type. You never get tomato, squash, and carrot seeds in the same packet! Not only does each type of seed have different sunshine, moisture, and seed depth requirements, mixing the types of seeds you plant makes weed removal and eventual harvest more difficult. What type of seeds are you planting?

If during the 1940s and 1950s the train industry had recognized that it was in the transportation business, and not the train business, it wouldn't have suffered so greatly at the hands of the airline industry. Max Factor observes that his cosmetics are merely chemicals when they leave the factory, but when purchased in a department store, they represent hope. Because their entire focus is on the adjustment, many chiropractors think that's what they're selling. But few patients want adjustments. It's merely the means by which you deliver what patients really want. If patients could get what they wanted some other way, they would. In fact, don't many patients try other methods *before* consulting your office?

If patients don't want adjustments per se, what do they want? Pain relief? Sure. Avoid surgery? Sure. Stop taking pain pills and muscle relaxers? Sure. The list goes on. To the dismay of many doctors, few patients enter the office with the goal of improving their posture, range of motion, kyphotic curve, or avoiding the degenerative effects of uncorrected spinal trauma. Few patients want true health–most just want to get through life with as little pain as possible. So, what business are you in?

Depends what type of seeds you're planting. Don't plant radish seeds if you want beans!

If you've ever had a garden or tried to raise a few tomatoes in a window box, you've already learned one important lesson when it comes to growing things: you can't rush or speed up the process. There are no shortcuts. You can tell the amateur "green thumbs" immediately. Like children, whose sense of time is distorted, many beginning gardeners are constantly checking the ground for the first green sprout. For many, it's tempting to dig up a few seeds to see if they've germinated, sacrificing the potential bound up in the seed. Our instant gratification society has changed our expectations and made most of us too impatient. That first week to ten days tests the faith of many gardeners.

Did I say faith? Yes, there is an element of faith required. After preparing the soil, picking the right seeds, adding the proper amount of moisture, and making all the necessary preparations, one must have faith. If you lack faith, don't become a gardener! Faith is the belief in things unseen. You must have faith that if tended properly the seeds will germinate. Do you have the faith necessary to trust the inborn potential of each patient to be healthy?

If you must control everything, you may be inclined to force the seeds you've planted to grow on your terms instead of the blueprint programmed into them. You may unreasonably expect them to grow during the dead of winter or in the dark shade of a tree. Or you may neglect them, forgetting to water or weed. Growth occurs by a set of established principles–not by the gardener's rules or desires.

Think of your practice as a garden. What are the principles that govern practice growth? Even if you don't want the prize-winning produce needed to compete at the state fair, here are some ideas to keep in mind as you tend your garden practice.

Seeds: The seeds you sow will determine the crop you reap. If you want children and families interested in a long term chiropractic lifestyle, advertising in just about any form may be the wrong type of seeds. If you want responsible, cash-paying wellness patients, you won't get them by making the "deal of the week" or pandering to the outdated insurance mentality. If you want a harvest of patients that respect you and comply with your recommendations, be sure you're saying and doing the things that these types of patients respect and can act on. The seeds of your practice are the vision and purpose you see for yourself. Just as seeds contain the genetic encoding and the potential to produce a rutabaga or a cabbage, each patient has the potential, through the referral process to replicate another patient like themselves.

Soil: The soil required in your office is a healthy environment that can nurture seed (patient) growth. It is the "tone" of your office. Is it disorganized, stressful, pathologically neat, cluttered, unfocused, absent-minded, out of date, or unclear of its purpose? Does the staff work as a team? Are patients an interruption or the enemy? Is it easy to find parking? Are clinical procedures and financial policies in place that work? Soil, with the proper nutrients and stones or other obstacles removed, is essential for practice growth. It takes time to condition the soil, till it, and prepare it for planting. And it must be maintained. Fertilizer, crop rotation, and letting the ground lay fallow for a season is all part of the plan. Taking out, without putting back, upsets the natural balance of things. Today, more and more practitioners are recognizing that they took and took from their practices during the insurance era. Now they are realizing that they must reinvest in their practices and replace the depleted soil that was abused for years.

Sunshine: With the exception of mushrooms, rare fish, and certain insects found in the depths of caves, very little grows in the dark. It's the same with patients who are kept in the dark about chiropractic. While plants use chlorophyll to convert sunlight into energy, patients use your educational efforts to convert their experience of chiropractic into something they can tell others about. Just as the sun rises each day, broaden and expand the patients' understanding of how their bodies function and how chiropractic fits into their lives on every visit. Neglect this important illumination and you rob each seed of its full potential. Patients whither and become susceptible to the influence of skeptics and others who mistrust the body's inborn healing powers.

Water: Moisture, at the proper time and in the correct quantity and quality is another essential ingredient to proper seed management. Remember how sweet the air smells after an afternoon shower? Adjusting the spine to improve the patient's form and function is quite similar. Knowing when, where, and how much is the art of chiropractic. Too much water and the plant dies. Too little water and the plant becomes stunted and wilts.

Enemies: Without interference, the checks and balances of nature operate perfectly. Invading insects or hungry birds can make a quick breakfast of your seeds or your harvest. Weeds can steal nutrients from the soil. Taking reasonable precautions to avoid these threats is essential. Same with patients. As your patients blossom with renewed health, consider the enemies! Be alert to your attitudes about new patients as they simply become part of the expected office volume. Monitor procedures and policies that discourage nonsymptomatic care. A personality (or lack of one) that interferes with patient rapport or an office environment that is drab, uninteresting, and tired, are subtle worms and infections. They are rarely spoken of by patients and even more rarely acknowledged by chiropractors who are primarily focused on the delivery of adjustments.

Pruning: Like disciplining a child, pruning improves the quality of the fruit at harvest time. Any doctor who has ever asked a patient to leave the practice or has referred a patient down the street, already knows the value of pruning the practice. Yet pruning your practice needn't involve the confrontation of kicking patients out! An easier method is to slowly orient your procedures and policies so they attract and nurture the types of patients you especially enjoy serving. Examine your office hours, your willingness to accept assignment, office location, wellness care policies, what you charge families, the mark up on your X-rays, and the hundreds of other innocuous details that, when combined, shape the patient profile of your office. Make sure the seeds you want to grow can thrive in the soil you've prepared.

Harvest: Based on the seeds you plant, your harvest can vary. Have you been planting high yield personal injury seeds? Or seeds that produce a stable family practice? Maybe a hybrid seedless variety of workers comp cases that have difficulty reproducing? Until you can clearly visualize the outcome you want at harvest time, it is difficult to have enough courage and faith (there's that word again!) to institute the changes you want. Being able to hold that idea in your mind long enough and communicate it consistently enough to your staff and patients is a sizable challenge. And the glacial speed with which these changes often occur can discourage even the most ardent crusader. Persistence is required.

The harvest is a reflection of the seed. The garden is a reflection of the gardener. What are you growing? ■

IN SEARCH OF WATER

Throughout the Midwest, America's breadbasket, the water table is dropping. Wells that were dug years ago with 20 or 50 feet of water are dropping precipitously each year. At the current pace, many wells will dry up leaving municipalities, grain producers, and livestock ranchers without the essential ingredient to grow and feed the world.

Like chiropractic.

The assistance offered patients by insurance equality has diminished. Insurance companies are businesses, not a public utility, and have sent deductibles soaring and the number of people who can afford insurance coverage plummeting. The third party payer "water table" is dropping.

In the 1980s almost every chiropractor quickly aligned their practice to exploit the $100 deductibles and the willingness of the baby boom generation to give "alternative medicine" a try. Computers, staffing, and management procedures were employed to take advantage of this source of easy money. Instead of taking the weekend off, doctors and their staff would crowd hotel ballrooms to learn the proper codes, latest strategies, and most efficient procedures to extract money from insurance companies. Many offices accepted assignment to make this cash conduit as direct as possible. If the biblical principle that "your heart is where your money is," was any indication, worshiping at the golden ox of the insurance industry was the major concern of many offices.

After years of incorporating this arrangement, it almost seemed normal. For doctors who began practice in this era, the notion that one can practice *without* third party pay is a foreign idea difficult to understand. As the water table drops, all too many offices are getting caught at the high water mark, responding too slowly to the changing insurance environment. As the submersible pump brings up more air and sediment, be careful of the several knee-jerk reactions that may delay an effective response:

Defective equipment: Is the pump in good condition? Does it just need some repair? This is the response of doctors who start questioning their technique or even whether chiropractic works. As the practice wavers it's tempting to consult, conduct a seminar, or sell out to insurance companies to do "peer" reviews. Staff members are taught to use increasingly confrontive tactics on the phone to release money from insurance companies. Practicing seems less fun than before.

Drill deeper: If the water table is dropping, then drill the well even deeper, reason many. Either doctors decide to do what used to work with even more energy, or they look for ways to squeeze more out of inactive files. These are the doctors who see the artifacts of their twelve years of practice (hundreds of inactive files with brightly colored labels), and wonder how to reactivate them. For many practices you'd just as well buy a mailing list of strangers. The opportunity to educate, inspire, and lead all those patients into a bigger meaning of chiropractic and true health was squandered in an attempt to get still more new patients with $100 deductibles. Too bad.

Rain makers: As practice income drops and your highly-leveraged lifestyle of the 80s is endangered, the flimflam man with the drums and secret "rain dance" starts to look attractive. Trying to find the perfect practice management firm with the bold new ideas necessary to take your practice into the insurance-free decade of the 90s is an oxymoron, because most are still beating the dead horse of CPT codes and proper form completion, or teaching the value of FAX machines and electronic filing! Ultimately, what many doctors realize is that they didn't get a practice management firm when they signed on, they hired an *insurance* management firm. Know anyone who wants a buggy whip franchise or a washboard reconditioning factory?

Active prospecting: A common response is to simply drill some new wells. Suddenly rehab centers, water purifiers, and pyramid schemes to sell everything from vitamins to herbal shampoo, look attractive to chiropractors. Still others are looking around for states with the easiest licensing reciprocity to move to. And while disrupting your life and starting over may sound exciting, you're only prolonging the inevitable. It's just a matter of time.

Hoarding resources: Remember the discovery that Mr. Environmentalist, John Denver, had been found stashing gasoline in two big tanks at his Aspen compound? Hoarding doesn't work. And being afraid of the doctor who moves in down the street, thinking that he or she is going to "steal" your patients or that there aren't enough patients to go around is just wrong. In fact, if everyone in your community knew what you did and understood the value of what you do, there would be a line in front of your door!

If any of these metaphors strike home, here are some suggestions to start turning your practice around and acknowledging this new practice reality. Wishful thinking and denial are simply delaying tactics that will make the necessary changes even more difficult and painful. How bad does it have to get before you'll be prompted to abandon the status quo?

Conservation: Waste is out. Conservation is in. A lower overhead, combined with long-range thinking is essential. Have you visualized your practice one year and five years into the future? You must. Like your patients who are paying off their credit cards and avoiding the temptation of instant gratification, this is probably not the time to assume massive amounts of debt. Continue to reinvest in your infrastructure, but take a conservative approach and look for methods to decrease your expenses in ways that don't compromise patient care or patient perceptions of your office.

Rationing: When you pay $6,000 a year to a management firm for professional advice, no one is going to tell you about downward mobility. Some might think it's not "motivational." Start examining your personal and professional life. Just because you're a doctor, nobody "owes" you a living, a Mercedes, or a 6,000 square foot home. Make your practice and your lifestyle relevant to the times. Batten down the hatches and fasten your seat belts. Get out of debt and put a rein on the flashy and extravagant purchases that fuel your ego.

Recycling: The disposable world is gone. Think of each new patient as a potential lifetime friend–not a short term financial gain. Return to the family doctor idea that we all had when we were growing up. It's not just enough to get new patients, you have to learn ways of keeping them. Patient education, affordable fees, and convenient hours are more important than ever. Are you helping your patients place the appropriate value on chiropractic in the context of other financial and time demands?

Efficiency: Would you pay $12 for an equal number of minutes on your intersegmental table? Why do you think cash-paying patients will, or the increasingly rare insurance company should? Streamlining your practice by eliminating unimportant or distracting procedures is crucial. For many that could mean disengaging from the insurance industry altogether by no longer accepting assignment and rethinking the need for your computer and its associated overhead. Avoid opportunity chasing. Get focused. What's your purpose?

Actually this is an exciting time for chiropractic. Unfortunately, the easy money from abundant insurance policies kept a lot of marginal chiropractors in business. It attracted many to the profession for the wrong motives. The impending "shake out" will be cleansing and ultimately good for chiropractic and for patients.

The glass is half full. ∎

NO BRAKES

Ever remember starting your car and driving off, thinking the car was underpowered or not working properly? You felt silly later when you discovered the parking brake was still on! When you released the brake, the car glided effortlessly through traffic. Many practices are being operated with the brakes on, preventing the normal growth and fulfillment deserved by the doctor and staff.

If there was a big lever in the X-ray room, or a handle on some sort of control panel in the hallway closet, detecting and correcting an improper use of the brakes in your office would be easy and instantly obvious to anyone. There would be little need for seminars, consultants, or self-help books. Since these levers are hidden, hotel meeting room facilities, seminar speakers, motivational cassette manufacturers, and book publishers have a rosy future.

After consulting with countless doctors, touring their offices, and listening to still others on the telephone, I have developed a "lever map" of common lever locations in a chiropractic office. If your practice seems to be cruising with an unseen force holding it back, you might check the following locations:

Doctor's chiropractic philosophy: Chiropractic is poised to tap into the natural demand of wellness care. More and more of us are recognizing that the disease processes that threaten us most, are lifestyle influenced. A pervasive interest in diet, exercise, and mental attitude have captured the attention of late night televised "infomercials" that offer everything from permanent weight loss to the health secrets of dried foods. Chiropractors who have confined their chiropractic influence to the narrow domain of the relief of low back pain or the easiest personal injury cases will find their practice increasingly stressful. Frustrated medics who think that symptomatic relief is the only worthy dimension of chiropractic will find their practices implode upon them. Wellness is the growth market. Pain-relief-only puts the brakes on.

Doctor's physical conditioning: There may be nothing more pathetic than a doctor who wants to rise above his or her current patient volume, but doesn't have the energy to do anything more than merely survive. I have little sympathy for doctors who prefer gimmicks or get-rich-quick new patient schemes, to the more effective process of working on themselves. I'm not talking about narcissistic mirror watching! Until you have the mental discipline to accomplish the appropriate house cleaning on yourself, don't expect patients to respect you, comply with your recommendations, or refer others. If the insurance era of low deductibles made you lazy or gave you a "I'm-a-doctor-I-deserve-it" attitude, welcome to the 1990s. What have you done for us lately? Are you setting a good example? Are you healthy yourself?

Doctor's willingness to risk rejection: The fear of rejection is one of the most prevalent and powerful fears we face. It stops perfectly capable doctors from doing lectures, confronting patients to pay their bills, calling new patients after the first adjustment, asking for referrals, and the other countless proven techniques for growing a practice. "That's not me," they say on the telephone. "I just can't see myself doing that," they observe at a seminar. "Give me something else I can do to increase the size of my practice." When this fear is exhibited in salespeople it is referred to as "call reluctance." Observe the coffee shop clientele at 10 AM on a Monday morning. Staring into their coffee cups are the commissioned sales force that will have to make countless cold calls that week and risk rejection. Every one of them knows it's a numbers game. The more calls they make the more they will succeed. Yet, it is so easy to take a stranger's

"NO!" or a patient's blank stare personally. It's the doctor who can see beyond rejection that enjoys a brake-free practice.

Doctor's enthusiasm: After frequent seminars and rah-rahs in the hotel ballrooms at practice management groups, it's easy to forget that the world doesn't care. The world doesn't care about your practice. The world doesn't care about chiropractic. The world doesn't owe you a living. The only way you are granted a living, and chiropractic matters, is when you make it matter to those you encounter. If you're not excited about chiropractic, don't expect patients or anyone else to be either. Your ability to focus your energy and mental abilities to project the mystery and awe about chiropractic, is in direct proportion to the success you'll enjoy. Excitement and confidence, even when they're difficult to produce, are essential characteristics of the practitioner who has released the brakes.

Staff motivation: Doctors with low confrontational skills frequently trip over this lever. Worse than the fact that many offices are over-staffed, many continue to employ people whose foot dragging is more effective than anti-lock brakes! Have a friend call your office and attempt to become a new patient 20 minutes before closing time. Listen to the staff when a patient calls to cancel an appointment. Notice the way staff members back their cars into their parking spaces for a quick getaway at lunch or the end of the day. It's human nature to minimize the amount of work we do and avoid confrontation. What's the staff motivation to double the size of the practice? Or even to increase it 20%? Until you share a vision for the practice that inspires the staff and prompts them to invest their emotional currency, expect high turnover and petty bickering. Only when staff members truly perceive themselves as a part of your health care team, have an influence in the direction of the practice, are unafraid of the doctor, and are not kept in constant fear of losing their jobs, will you have a motivated staff. If you're going slow, maybe you should check to see if you're carrying the weight of unnecessary passengers.

Office layout: Funny how we're more willing to regularly update the model of car we drive than make changes to the office environment. New car purchases are easy to justify—new safety features, the new CD music entertainment center, better gas mileage, etc. Suggest changes in the office layout and you'd think B. J. had personally anointed each 10' X 10' fluorescently lit adjusting room. Make some changes! Even if all you do is replicate the Hawthorn Effect (increasing or decreasing the lighting in a factory resulted in increased production), changing your environment will result in improved productivity. Notions about doors on rooms, privacy, open offices, gowning patients, time spent with the patient, and all the other dogma and bigotry, has slowed down more practitioners than all the HMOs in town. Keep in mind countless patients are getting perfectly good results (and loving it), at the hands of doctors using the exact opposite procedure, technique, or office layout that you "believe" in! Their impact is greater because when it comes to office layout, they've been willing to try the second and third "right answer" not just the first answer that seemed to work years ago when they were a struggling cost-conscious new doctor.

Patient communications: Patient education is a favorite subject of mine, so you already know how important I think good patient communications are. It's one of those topics that prompts doctors to say, "Yeah, but what else do you have?" Those with brake-free practices recognize that the real day-to-day joy isn't how many new patients they get or how much money they make. It's enjoying the process of "cracking the safe." The safe is each patient's cerebral cortex. Every patient has a different combination. Without access to the safe there is poor rapport, poor compliance, and few referrals. Find the combination, and the dance you dance with each patient is a lot more interesting and fulfilling. Until you enjoy the process of finding the combination you'll never achieve "passing-lane" speed. Get out the sandpaper and rough up those fingers! Listen carefully for the tumblers to fall. Pay attention to what it will take to help each individual patient "get it."

Notice that none of these suggestions rely on the cooperation of the weather, the size of your town, medical referrals, or changes in the trend towards managed care. *You* are in charge. It's your responsibility to find the brake lever and release it. These suggestions may not be as exciting as going into debt for a new-fangled this or a high-tech that, but then brakes are pretty simple devices. They create friction. Reducing the friction frees up energy for more productive pursuits.

I live in Colorado Springs where the Great Plains meet the Rocky Mountains. The city is situated at the foot of Pikes Peak. Tourists from around the world come to Colorado Springs to drive to the peak's 14,000 foot summit. On a clear day you can see forever. Car rental companies at the airport regularly remind "flatlanders" how to drive in the mountains, particularly how to properly handle the descent of Pikes Peak. Even so, a favorite summer afternoon pastime among gift shops at the foot of the Pikes Peak Highway is to count the number of cars with their back tires on fire from using their brakes for 12 miles instead of shifting into a lower gear!

Is your practice on fire, or is that just your brakes I smell? ■

SHOP AND COMPARE

During the late 1970s and 1980s there was a large furniture store in town that used the phrase, "Shop and Compare" in all its advertising. The constant stream of TV commercials aimed at the sizable transient military community in town, featured the thick accent of the store's owner. The store is out of business today, apparently the result of more and more shoppers taking the store's advice! The skill of properly comparing is a valuable talent we learn at an early age. It helps us determine what we like, better differentiate physical spaces, the passage of time, and relative speed. Comparing one thing with another helps us to define our reality. This is a two-edged sword. Those who feel compelled to "keep up with the Joneses" or are disenchanted with their noses, breasts, hair (or lack of it), have fallen into this trap and become prisoners of comparing themselves to others or to the "norm."

"Why do kids look into the bathroom stall when I'm going to the bathroom at school," asked my 8-year old son out of the blue one day. I didn't tell him that the reason was the same as why high school boys take split-second glances at each other in the shower after gym class. But I did explain that it's because many of us need reassurance that we are like others. It is somehow comforting to know that others share our same fears, concerns, sizes, or shapes. This desire to fit in explains all kinds of bizarre behavior—everything from inhaling toxic fumes from the low temperature burning of tobacco, to piercing various body parts so decorative metal can be inserted. Gangs, cults, and other non-mainstream social groups gain their strength by using the com-

197

parative differences between "us" and "them" to offer those so persuaded that they "belong" to something, regardless of how destructive it is.

Doctors compare themselves with other doctors. They compare practices. They compare the physical trappings of success. They compare statistics. They compare the things that are the easiest to see, yet overlook the peace of mind, spiritual health, family relationships, and "fun quotients" that are more accurate measurements of one's true success.

"It's not fair. We're always available for our patients, we're always trying to improve our practice, and we're conscious of trying to say and do the right things, but the office down the street seems busier than ours," lamented a doctor over dinner one night. Apparently, after five or six years of struggling, the couple was still feeling the pinch from undercapitalization and the pressure of comparing themselves to others. In fact, upon further discussion it was revealed that they didn't even respect the doctor in the office down the street—yet they were comparing themselves with him! They seemed to overlook the beautiful home they were living in, their two respectful and well adjusted teenagers, the valuable healing skills they had, their friends, their health, and their tremendous potential for the future.

If you always look for flaws, shortcomings, or inadequacies, you'll find them. Only one person was perfect, and they crucified him. Lighten up!

When we compare things we tend to compare new situations with previously related things. If there is a huge difference between what we expect or have stored in our memory, our first response is to question our sense organs. If, after we rub our eyes and take an inventory of our faculties and we still see the same thing, we become intensely interested and often have a heightened sense of concentration. Wouldn't it be nice if patients were in this state during your report of findings?

Patients are continually comparing their chiropractic experiences in your office with their experiences elsewhere. The medical benchmark normally used, creates some interesting conflicts for the patient if the doctor is unaware how disorienting certain aspects of chiropractic can be.

Treatment on first visit: Patients are accustomed to a one-visit experience with a health care provider. They expect something to happen, a prescription, a recommendation to discontinue some activity, or some other guidance. When you examine your patients and send them packing after the first visit without even an ice pack or directions for self-care, patients feel cheated, especially after paying for the examination and a series of X-rays that are held hostage until a subsequent visit. If you are adamant about withholding the adjustment until future visits, you must make sure you address this issue and clearly explain why. Otherwise, when patients compare their experience in your office with interactions with other doctors, they are likely to assume you're holding back information or enjoy this cruel power ploy.

One visit treatment: The medical profession has taught today's patient that the drug they need or the procedure required should only take one visit. Continued visits recommended over weeks or months sounds suspicious. "If my problem didn't show up until I bent over funny last week, why am I going to need three months worth of Initial Intensive Care," reasons the ill-informed patient. This patient attitude is especially common if you're educating your patients with the bone-out-of-place model of chiropractic. Without a broader explanation of the muscle and soft tissue involvement, patients figure it should take about one visit to put a bone back into the right place. Maybe two or three visits tops–if you're not very good!

Waiting time: Again, most patients look to the medical community for guidelines as to how long they should have to wait in the reception room. During the early stages of care, waiting twenty to thirty minutes for their appointment is endured. As they learn that frequent visits over a long period of time will be required, running on schedule is extremely important. As patients start feeling better they find it increasingly hard to justify the cost, in terms of time, of following the doctor's recommendations. And it's not just the time in the reception room, it's the total elapsed time of the office visit for a procedure that often takes only three or four minutes to complete.

Office environment: This is an aspect of comparison that many chiropractic doctors overlook as they create an office that pretty much looks like a medical practitioner's office. And while this may serve to put new chiropractic patients at ease, it can undermine a patient's long term compliance. Who would want to visit the environment of a medical doctor's office again and again and again? A chiropractic office that wants to develop long term client relationships needs to look contemporary, reflect ergonomical awareness, invite children, be creative, interesting, and ever changing. It must be a testimonial of what patients with a more normally functioning nervous system want—stimulation.

Nurse/Chiropractic Assistant: Chiropractic patients who perceive the doctor as too busy or unapproachable often find themselves asking the staff questions about their health or chiropractic issues. This seems to happen more frequently in offices that have the good fortune of low staff turnover in which chiropractic assistants project confidence in their daily duties. Many patients are alarmed to find that the staff hasn't received any formal training like their equivalent in the medical arena. While many states are addressing this issue, particularly in the X-ray technology area, it suggests how important it is to display not just the doctor's diplomas, but those of the staff. Take the effort to frame and display staff certificates for seminar training and other continuing education.

Patient responsibility: I think this issue is the most fundamental. In medicine, the responsibility for healing is on the doctor doing the surgery or administering the right drugs. In a chiropractic setting, the patient is constantly reminded that healing is the responsibility of the patient. This is the primary difference that can produce a participative, involved chiropractic patient or a skeptical, noncompliant chiropractic patient. A patient's willingness to accept responsibility for poor habits, spinal neglect, and the need to learn more about true health is a good indicator of the prognosis. When chiropractic doctors show too much enthusiasm to accept a new patient or too willingly allow the patient to dictate terms of the doctor/patient relationship, it usually interferes with the patient's perception of responsibility. Doctors with the courage and discipline to confront each patient on these issues enjoy better compliance and satisfaction.

Anticipating, acknowledging, or pointing out these obvious and sometimes subtle comparative differences can enhance patient rapport. Ignoring them invites disappointment or apprehension.

Be careful who and what you compare yourself with. The survival of chiropractic is better assured by acknowledging and embracing the differences between chiropractic and medicine. Trying to be like medical doctors is not a guarantee of acceptance. Ultimately, the future holds the most promise for those doctors who are the least "full of themselves" so they can be sensitive to the expectations of their patients. ■

WISH YOU WERE HERE

Doctors who enjoyed the giddy ride of insurance in the 1980s have rows and rows of files that are souvenirs of this bygone era. These serve as a constant reminder to what could have been–the pain relief patients who could have bloomed into long-term clients. The husband that could have inspired a spouse. The mom who could have influenced an entire family to begin care. There are those doctors and staff members who still remember the names and faces connected to these files. Because they do, they think they are "worth" more than they really are. They think there is "hidden gold" in those files. When attempting to sell a practice, these tangible reminders are often overvalued by those who created the files. Sadly, these are often remnants of what was, rather than what can be.

Some of those patients are angry because chiropractic didn't work. Some of those patients had their problem "fixed" and don't see a need to ever return. Most did not receive even a fundamental chiropractic education, stunting their growth from patients into clients. The unfortunate result is that most of the X-rays in those files would be more valuable as a source of silver than as the groundwork for reactivating patients!

After being hounded by an aggressive recall program, few patients feel comfortable returning to your office for fear the inevitable "I told you so" might accompany the consultation. Still others, so put off by the high pressure recall attempts, are prompted to enroll in the federal witness protection plan or simply vow never to return–even if the symptoms do.

Interestingly, few doctors know exactly why their patients drop out of care. Without this knowledge, most offices are powerless to prevent it. If you knew why your patients dropped out of care, you could take steps to avoid it. Oh, there are theories and conjecture that successfully protect the ego of the doctor, however few doctors know why *their* patients discontinue care. In fact, this phenomenon is given a special name; premature dismissal. Not only does this term make it easy to shift the blame, it obscures the fact that the patient fired you!

When getting more new patients to replace the ones that fired you was easier, this symptom was overlooked. Today, as bragging rights about one's patient retention statistics become more important than new patient volume, this can no longer be ignored. Without receiving a pink slip with the specific reason(s) listed, a high-powered recall script delivered by a reluctant staff person seems like the only solution.

Has your recall program ever created a chiropractic client?

My work with patient focus groups has revealed two of the most frequent reasons patients leave the practice after getting satisfactory relief of their symptoms. Plug these two holes and watch the number of cash paying families seeking preventive chiropractic care increase.

1. Can't afford to continue. This is the number one reason why patients drop out of care. And it's not because they don't have the money. These are the same patients who never miss a winter ski trip to Vail or snorkeling in Hawaii and drive off in their BMW. This is the excuse patients use when they don't put the same "value" the doctor places on chiropractic care. Helping patients place the proper value on their chiropractic care is one of the most important unspoken responsibilities doctors have.

There are two choices for doctors who want more patients to enjoy nonsymptomatic care: lower the price of wellness care or add more "value" to the chiropractic experience. Lowering the cost of care is the easiest and most frequently chosen method. Doctors simply provide two different types of care, sickness care and wellness care and offer two different fees. If it is legal in your state, it may solve the problem, yet usually only attract those already predisposed to a preventive approach to health: the regular teeth flossers and seat belt wearers. Many of these are the same patients who would come in once a month anyway, but with a lower price, show up more frequently.

Adding value takes more energy, creativity, and resources. Something besides obvious symptoms must motivate patients to return to your office and pay cash out of their own pocket. Some ways doctors add value is to help raise each patient's self esteem, create an interesting and creative environment, keep waiting times to a minimum, have an attractive personality, implement consistent patient education, and enhance other "intangibles" about the office visit and their chiropractic "performance."

2. See no need to continue. This is a warning sign that you didn't educate the patient sufficiently or didn't make chiropractic care relevant to their lifestyle. With insurance gone, this is more important than ever. While there is plenty written about the why, how, when, and where of patient education, the challenge here is the faith required by doctors to trust that the energy they expend in educating patients will be returned in the form of higher patient visit retention. The lack of guarantees or any form of instant gratification thwarts many doctors from taking the effort to help each patient "get it." Instead, many offices go after the "easy" patients; the personal injury cases, worker's compensation injuries, and patients who work for companies that still have generous insurance benefits. A recurring fantasy for all too many doctors is becoming a chiropractic consultant or company chiropractor for a major business down the street.

This is the same old rationale that doctors use to convince themselves that if they just had enough new patients, all their problems would be solved. If you're tempted to make this argument, count the number of inactive files you're storing. You've already *had* enough new patients! They're just not staying. Which brings us back to the importance of patient education.

If you're inclined to attempt to use some type of reactivation letter to bring back the patients lurking in those files, be sure your letter addresses these two major points. Perhaps something like this:

Dear (Dropped Out Patient)

At a recent staff meeting, your name came up. We noticed it's been a while since we've seen you and we were wondering how you were doing.

Many of the health complaints we see in adult cases are often the result of many years of overlooked spinal problems. Even after the pain or other symptoms are gone, underlying muscle and soft tissue damage predispose many patients to a relapse.

That's why many of our patients decide to continue with some type of ongoing maintenance/wellness care, even though they feel better. In fact, we now have a special program that makes this type of preventive care very affordable. Call or drop by the office for more details.

If you're doing great, congratulations! It's always nice to be reminded how well chiropractic works. When you need a little "tune-up" or you want to help prevent future problems, we'll be here to help.

Best regards,

Dr. (Your Name Here)

Make sure you address the two primary issues of cost (value) and patient education. While for many patients, learning about soft tissue involvement at this stage may be too late, including it helps justify your concern.

Getting patients to return to the office to benefit from wellness chiropractic care is difficult. It is more likely they'll make the transition as part of their normal reduction in visit frequency. In other words, it's easier to keep the patient, than to get them to reactivate themselves on a nonsymptomatic basis. Wait for a relapse or change your patient education strategy, office fee policy, or help the patient perceive more value in their care. Otherwise, you're likely to get postcards from patients enjoying their exotic vacations who write, "wish you were here." ∎

CREATING TANGIBLE ARTIFACTS

The risk of selecting the "wrong" doctor, lawyer, CPA, or other licensed professional can be quite high. Malpractice, legal oversights, missing a filing deadline, wrong diagnosis, and other dangers lurk behind yellow page ads, direct mail offers, and mall show hucksters of virtually all licensed professionals. Each of these services is intangible—the consumer doesn't know for sure if the quality of the service is good or bad until after committing to, and receiving, the service. Unlike a pair of pants, car tires, or other tangible items, professional services like chiropractic cannot be tested or tried in advance. This intangibility factor makes picking the right chiropractic doctor difficult for a new patient, even with the reassurances of a referring friend. This is just one of several reasons why you should have an office brochure. Evaluate your current office brochure or your need to create one by these four criteria:

1. Tangible artifact. An office brochure can represent the quality of care the patient is likely to encounter in your office. Patients use your office brochure (building exterior, office furnishings, business card, etc.) and other physical manifestations as a representation of your attention to detail. If your brochure is printed in one color on cheap paper without pictures or illustrations, patients can draw the likely conclusion that you're new, short of cash, not very successful, don't intend to be in practice long, or just aren't very observant. Any one of these issues can have an adverse effect on a patient's level of trust and confidence in you. In many ways a poor office brochure can do more harm than not having one! Without an office brochure, patients may depend upon a prestigious address, staff phone manners, or other symbols of the quality of your care. With a low quality brochure you broadcast your lack of attention to detail or lack of success. If you can't do it right, it's best not to do one at all!

2. Remove internal dialogue. You may be oblivious to it, but the media has made most new patients quite apprehensive about selecting a non-traditional, alternative form of healing. While this is slowly changing, many of today's typical new patients bring with them many myths and misconceptions about you, your profession, and their own judgment for even considering consulting your office. If you recognize the noisy internal dialogue these notions create, you can address many of them in your office brochure. Explain your educational achievements, the safety of adjustments, availability of affordable financial arrangements, and that "how long you decide to benefit from chiropractic care is always up to you." Patients reason that a doctor sensitive enough and confident enough to recognize and volunteer information about these issues must be good. Offer information about these and other issues and watch new patient rapport improve.

3. Outreach vehicle. What's especially valuable about an office brochure is that it can go places that you may never get to go. When used as a first visit handout it can serve as a referral tool. When mailed to a 3-5 mile radius of your office, it can plant seeds and perhaps prompt those sitting on the fence to take action. Your office brochure can be a new patient ambassador for your office. Let the world know it exists, so requesting a copy of it can provide a low commitment action step for someone considering chiropractic care. "Not ready to start care? Request a copy of our office brochure that explains chiropractic and what we do to help patients regain their health."

4. Consistent explanations. Doctors who have found a typographical error in their newsletter know the permanence of a printed mistake. Of course the reverse is true, too. Once you get your unique approach to chiropractic finalized in your brochure, it's the same explanation wherever the brochure goes. If you depend solely on your current patient's ability to describe what you do, then you already know why it's hard for them to get their friends and family to start care! Sadly, even your best patients find it difficult to explain chiropractic in terms that are informative, much less motivational! Equip them with a tool to explain and defend their decision to others. How do you want chiropractic described to the world?

Clearly, your office could probably benefit from a high quality brochure. Before you commit the time and energy to create and produce one, make sure you have some clearly defined uses for it. Taking delivery of boxes of your brand new brochure is not the time to figure out what you're going to do with it! Here are some suggestions for possible uses:

1. Direct mail. Design your brochure so a bulk rate permit can be printed or stamped on it along with an address label. Plan on mailing it periodically, perhaps as often as several times a year! Frequency is the key.

2. Current patient handout. Use it to stimulate referrals by presenting a copy to every patient on about the tenth visit or so when your patients can clearly ascertain that chiropractic works. "Hey, if the subject of chiropractic ever comes up at work, here's our brochure that explains what we do."

3. Prospective new patient kit. Use your clinic brochure as the cornerstone to a new patient kit. Include copies of research findings, explanations of chiropractic, and other handouts that could help anticipate and answer some of the questions a prospective patient might have about chiropractic. Perhaps advertise in your office brochure that this packet exists.

4. Rack brochure. If you invest in chiropractic brochures to help answer questions and stimulate referrals, make sure your office is represented in your brochure rack. This is a good argument for making your office brochure the size and shape that will fit in your reception room brochure rack and a #10 envelope.

5. Outside events. If you do screenings, lay lectures, speaking engagements, school programs, or other outreach events, make sure you have a "leave behind" that can prompt interested people to consult your office. Plant seeds that may not germinate for months or years. What's the hurry?

6. Professional referrals. Stimulate interest and awareness among other health and legal professionals who might be inclined to refer patients and clients your way. Include a copy of your office brochure with a cover letter explaining "...just wanted you to know that we're in the area and prepared to offer your patients (clients) the highest quality state-of-the-art chiropractic care..."

I'm sure there are other uses. The point is, know what you're going to do with your brochures *before* you order them so you can be sure to include the right kind of information. And what should your brochure say? Ironically, very little!

The most important ingredient in a successful office brochure is a lot of pictures. We are a visual culture (70% of the public can't remember what it was like before television). Watch yourself the next time you thumb through a magazine. First your eyes go to the picture. If the picture is interesting you study the picture then you look for a caption. If the photo caption is interesting you check out the accompanying story. Rule number one: use lots of pictures. Rule number two: tell your entire story with photo captions. Rule number three: keep the copy short.

Ideas for pictures might include the exterior of your building (if it's attractive), staff member greeting a new patient, the doctor consulting with a patient, setting up the patient for X-rays, giving a report of findings, in the adjusting room with a patient, the doctor working late at night at the desk, the doctor working with a child, sports injury, or other specialty; the list goes on. The key idea is to remove the fear of the unknown and address issues that prospective new patients are likely to have ("Do I have to take off my clothes?"). Your chiropractic philosophy? Put a little in, but keep it conventional and mainstream. Remember your readers are firmly entrenched in the germ theory and the treatment of symptoms! Don't scare them off by forcing them to wade through a lesson in deductive reasoning!

These basics should get you going. Work with a professional graphic design firm. Invest the extra money to print full color. Remember, you're making a tangible artifact that represents the quality of the chiropractic care you provide. It costs just as much to send a one color brochure through the mail as it does a well-designed four color brochure. The only difference is the impact it makes and the impression it leaves.

Perhaps a brochure seems like an expensive luxury. Or you feel paralyzed to begin because you've never done one before. Remember that the best offices have the best patient communications. Giving your practice tangibility can have some very tangible rewards–more new patients. ■

THE BUSINESS
OF BUSINESS CARDS

There are some doctors who gain solace from the notion that there appears to be an almost inverse relationship between one's business skills and one's healing talents. Since healing a patient's hurts is "more important," all too many doctors almost celebrate their poor business skills. The lack of a killer instinct when enticing a patient to begin care, or the tough-skinned firing of a staff member, is avoided at all costs. If one must revert to such savage interpersonal skills, then one must not be a very good healer, goes the logic. And while this isn't an endorsement for such Neanderthal business practices, thinking that being a businessperson and a compassionate healer occupy opposing sides of a coin is just not true. Being comfortable wearing both hats is not only fashionable, it's critical to one's success in the new practice environment of the 1990s.

This notion is especially apparent in the creation and distribution of a doctor's business card. It is such a small thing, normally 2" by 3 1/2", that it rarely gets the attention by management gurus that it should. It is often one of the first visible things created by a new doctor to be used to create the first (and most lasting) impression of those who receive one. While doctors may spend hundreds of dollars of their time and energy finding the perfect office location and hiring an attorney to review the office lease and then spend still thousands more on paint, carpet, and furnishings, the lowly business card is given 10 minutes of thought and costs just a few dollars to produce. Overlooking small details is a good way to sabotage a practice.

Why are business cards so important? Like an office brochure, they are a tangible (and portable) representation of your practice. While it may be just a small, rectangular piece of paper, a business card can be a powerful tool for growing your practice.

As I meet doctors at seminars and speaking engagements, I am stunned by the number of doctors who claim to own business cards, but don't seem to have them with them. Embarrassed, they pat their pockets, rifle through a veritable filing cabinet of a wallet, but come up empty. I think part of the problem is the printers who print business cards.

When you order your business cards they come in a cute little box. It's about the size of a large jewelry box, and it almost seems a shame to remove any. The weight of the paper, the smell of the ink, and the precision cutting of the cards that fit perfectly in the box, makes one hesitate before removing any cards from the set. A dozen or so cards are removed, placed in your wallet or purse and the rest of the box is put on the shelf, where all too often, they remain; a box of 500 cards lasting many doctors two, three or more years!

Part of the reluctance that doctors may have about getting rid of their business cards may be due in part to having had business cards shoved in their faces at conventions by aggressive computer software salesmen and headrest paper marketeers. Cleaning their pockets out and throwing away a handful of cards, obtained from "running the gauntlet" of a typical state association convention, can put one in the frame of mind that most cards are discarded (so to speak). How you treat business cards shouldn't be a judge of how others use business cards. Networking groups sponsored by the chamber of commerce are a good example of what a business card can do. The whole purpose of these groups is to find contacts in other businesses that might become potential customers.

If you'd rather not rub shoulders with the Realtors, seamless gutter providers, and insurance salesmen, that's all right. But what about the dry cleaners, car repairmen, and hair stylists? These and other types of service providers, who are in contact with countless others, are logical recipients of your business cards. Get into the habit of giving a card out frequently to these other professionals. Unfortunately, many doctors think that once they've given someone their card, that it automatically goes into a little binder of some kind in which duplicates are frequently removed. Probably not. Keep in mind as you give your cards away, that your card may be given to a third party you haven't even met yet. Make sure people who encounter and influence others have an ample supply of your cards!

A business card is merely a simple and inexpensive way to accurately supply your name, address, phone number, and other pertinent information about your practice. It can serve as a form of aided recall. "I know a great chiropractor. She's not like all the other chiropractors you've heard about. In fact, I have her card. Here. Call her."

What does a good business card look like? Your card should graphically represent you and your office. If yours is a formal office, perhaps your card should be more corporate looking. If yours is a place where children and families frequent, maybe the graphic approach should be "friendlier." The tone your card projects is affected by the thickness of the paper, color of the paper, color of the ink(s), typeface, and layout.

If you recognize the importance of rapidly depleting your supply of cards by generously giving them out to everyone you encounter, consider a variety of designs. Perhaps create a Monday card, a Tuesday card, etc. A different card for a different day of the week! Then when someone politely turns you down, having received a card from you the week before, "Oh, you must of gotten my Wednesday card. This is my Thursday card. I have a different card for every day of the week, because I just never know who I might run into that might need a chiropractic doctor." Have fun with it.

Probably the most overlooked opportunity of most practice business cards I see is the empty back side. For a profession that the general public misunderstands, it seems such a waste to ignore the blank surface on the back. If you don't use it for recording appointment dates and times, consider writing a short paragraph for the back side. Maybe the paragraph on the back of one card describes your chiropractic philosophy. Another might explain what happens on a new patient's typical first visit. Another might explode a common myth about chiropractic. The opportunity to provide quick, bite-sized, thought-provoking ideas are endless. The first step is to stop looking at your business cards in the old fashioned, white-paper-black-ink limited vision way!

While you're at it, if the idea is to get as many cards as possible out into your community, why not provide cards for your staff? The expense is small, and the prestige it gives your staff with their friends and family is enormous. Make sure they understand the idea is to get rid of as many cards as possible. They don't do any good sitting neatly in the box they come in.

Get your business card professionally designed. Interview some graphic designers and explain what kind of image you want your card(s) to project. Look at samples of other business cards and letterhead designs they've worked on. Find someone you think you'd like working with and get going. The design and production may cost a couple of hundred dollars (get a fixed bid in advance), but you'll be amazed at what can be done with seven square inches on the front and seven square inches on the back.

Your business card is a small thing. And changing it won't save your practice or solve a new patient problem. Yet, reevaluating your card and how you're using it can increase the exposure of your practice in subtle ways. Gimmicks that instantly put 50 new patients on your doorstep are just that, gimmicks. Taking a proactive role in letting the world know where you are and what you do is a way to attract patients in *quantities* you can handle with the *qualities* you enjoy serving. Which makes the *business* of chiropractic as enjoyable as the *healing* of chiropractic. ■

DO YOU BELIEVE?

I like to get the attention of chiropractic audiences by beginning my presentation, "Good morning. My name is Bill Esteb. I'm not a doctor of chiropractic, I'm not a chiropractic assistant, and I don't believe in chiropractic!"

After everyone gasps, and after a dramatic pause I continue, "I *know* in chiropractic."

The difference between knowing and believing is an interesting bifurcation point that separates today's chiropractors into two distinct groups. At either extreme in both groups you'll find successful doctors having fun. But closer to the middle of this continuum you'll find doctors struggling to maintain control of their practices and remain focused on chiropractic. They *believe* chiropractic works, but they want to *know* why. Living with this ambiguity is just too much for some.

The "knowers" are incessant readers. On the corner of their desktops you see the latest scientific journals, crammed with a sea of gray type and punctuated with occasional graphs and countless footnotes and references. This is the breakfast of champions for those of an analytical bent. Through their reading and ceaseless personal research, they confirm their clinical findings and look for the objective truths that govern physiology and pathology. Fearful that chiropractic or their particular approach may not be the very best for the patient, they continue their search for the chiropractic Holy Grail. Distracted by opinions and conclusions that run counter to their training or clinical experience, they practice in a twilight zone of

217

tentativeness. They avoid taking a stand or making definitive recommendations. Their lack of confidence is detected by patients, sabotaging compliance. The doctor's unwillingness to volunteer anything to a patient that can't be proven with at least two references in peer review journals can be perceived by patients as a poor attempt to disguise a grave condition! This creates a self-fulfilling prophecy that sucks the doctor further into the vortex of uncertainty.

If you don't want patients to merely *believe* in chiropractic (because you don't), at least allow them to believe in *you*!

Doctors wishing to escape this malaise are faced with several choices. One is simply to live with the ambiguity and forge on. This "fake-it-until-you-make-it" school of thought has helped many to move on to more important issues in their personal and professional growth. Another choice is to pull all the stops and begin an aggressive research program to get your questions answered. You may find your answers documented somewhere, or worse, you won't. The risk here is you'll have to make an even more uncomfortable decision if you get to the end of your crusade and come up empty handed. Of course another choice, and one that an increasing number of doctors have made, is to leave the healing arts for something more concrete, perhaps accounting or engineering.

At the other end of the spectrum are the "believers." These doctors have reduced chiropractic to a biomechanical philosophy. They are quick to point out that they don't heal the body, but unlock the inborn potential of patients to be healthy. "I don't diagnose and I don't treat disease." And they're absolutely correct. The only problem is, their patients don't know whether they should be praying or receive the "laying on of hands" or both. Patients leave the office unaccustomed to assuming so much responsibility for their own recovery and unsure they even consulted a doctor!

These doctors don't need proof that chiropractic works. They've seen it work for years. Having experienced their own personal brush with chiropractic that prompted them to investigate it as a first or second career, these doctors exude humility and a calm sense of confidence that patients find comforting. Yet, patients are frustrated that the doctor ignores their mention of symptomatic complaints. Like the holier-than-thou attitude projected by auto mechanics who ignore the owner's explanations or suggested cause of the "funny clicking sound," these doctors often refuse to acknowledge their patient's attempts at providing feedback. The result is a patient who gets well, but feels "unconnected" with the doctor.

The frustration these doctors face is the clash between their highly refined philosophy and their patient's lack of one. So while the doctor may be right, he or she often doesn't enjoy the rapport that other doctors do. Instead, practice is an endless battle to "reeducate" the masses. It requires massive amounts of energy and a total commitment to chiropractic. B. J.'s books are consulted regularly and quarterly get-togethers with other similarly inclined philosophers fuel the fires.

Both believers and knowers suffer from the new Scientism that has swept our culture. The scientific method has run wild, creating a generation that is suspicious of anything that can't be proved, measured, or observed with the five senses. With the advent of gene mapping, organ transplants, nuclear medicine, and other so-called "scientific" advances in medicine, Scientism may be one of the biggest barriers to the acceptance of chiropractic.

To combat this tide, it's interesting to note that a large percentage of today's most frequently encountered diseases and health complaints are the result of a lifetime of poor health habits. Science and technology offer little for cigarette smoking induced lung cancers, cholesterol-laden diet induced heart disease, or sedentary lifestyle induced non-specific health complaints. For many it will be too late when they discover the limitation of "scientific" health care in the reversal of a lifetime of poor decisions or a lack of discipline. There will be outrage at the misleading TV commercials "curing" this or that. Like Dorothy who sees the real Wizard of Oz operating the controls behind the curtains, the media and the public will be asking better questions. Disillusionment with medicine will create an important opportunity for chiropractic.

The fact is, more and more people are recognizing that the medical model doesn't work. The *New England Journal of Medicine* has observed what a growing number of chiropractic doctors already know: more and more people are consulting "alternative" forms of health professionals. The tide is turning.

The future of chiropractic is better assured by separating chiropractic from the medical arts. The time when many chiropractors are tired and just want to be accepted, happens to be the very time when it is crucial that the world know the difference. The solution is to give your patients enough science so they can believe. ■

THE ADVANTAGES OF UNITY

I think it was HUD Secretary Jack Kemp who said that you cannot have a democracy without morality. In other words, you can't have equality without shared values. Think about the drive by shootings, graffiti, ineffective public works projects, and the foreign aid that is wasted. The lack of shared values produces conflict and misunderstanding. This is not unlike the class warfare of the French Revolution or the caste system of India. Shared values are crucial for harmony, trust, and equality. Without this important common bond, discord and distracting infighting is produced.

Sounds like chiropractic.

Consider the damage done to the acceptance and utilization of chiropractic because of the continued straight/mixer fight. Count the cost of the ACA/ICA battles. Figure the distraction of the CCE/SCASCA wars. Try to measure the wasted energies of the philosophy/science debate, and the schism created by school politics and dogmatic adjusting techniques. The we/them battles of chiropractic have raged since the beginning. Just think how far we *could* have come in the last 100 years if the lack of shared values hadn't plagued this profession!

Consciously or not, there is a portion of the profession interested in destroying the other faction because of these issues. While this conflict rages as to who is more correct, take a look around. We have a profession in which doctors depend more on entrepreneurs for the latest information, instead of state chiropractic associations and societies. Notice the patchwork of state laws governing the scope of practice. Watch the huge insurance companies dividing and conquering offices. The profession lacks a centralized resource for chiropractic research information. Where's the fully supported and funded national public relations campaign? Where's the sharply focused national lobbying efforts? Why is there a general disinterest and apathy for the major political organizations? It is a testimonial to the power of chiropractic (as uniquely rendered by thousands of "Lone Rangers") that this profession has even survived!

You'd think with so many chiropractors getting such great results in their practices, that there would be something that everyone could rally around and claim as common ground. It seems that a good place to start is at the beginning with the original vision that chiropractic is a science, art, and philosophy. Is there any one of these three legs that a majority of chiropractors can agree on?

Philosophy

Probably not. The most pragmatic suggest that philosophy of any kind just isn't relevant for day to day living, much less in the business of chiropractic. So the notion of cause and effect, freeing the inborn abilities of the body to heal, and other philosophical tenets, seem for many, on the fringe, and too far out of the scientific mainstream. Too bad.

Art

With all the different adjusting styles, especially as low force and soft tissue work seems to be embraced by more and more doctors, the "art" of chiropractic is unlikely to be a major rallying point. Too many doctors define their very existence by the particular adjusting approach they've selected. "Everyone who uses the blasphemous XYZ technique should by shot!" reason all too many. Some use their hands, others don't. Some take three minutes, others take 20. Some adjust one bone, others the entire spine. Some restrict to just the spine, others adjust extremities too. Heck, there's some doctors who don't even adjust at all!

Guess the art of chiropractic is unlikely to be a rallying point.

Science

You'd think that something as objective as science would be specific enough that we could rally around *that*! Dean Edell, M.D., on his national call-in talk show about health, intoned what many in the other healing arts are thinking. If chiropractors are going to make claims at helping this or that, please bring forth the proof. Fair enough. The problem is, many can't even agree that a subluxation exists!

Seems to me the only way to see who is more correct is arm wrestling. Best two out of three wins.

Seriously, in other professions there are differences and strong personalities too. While there may be six different recognized approaches to removing an appendix or four major ways of performing a Caesarean section, most medical doctors seem less concerned about which method is used, as long as the intended results are safely achieved. Ah-hah! Can we agree on results?

Whether a patient gets results seems objective enough. Can we rally around the results of whatever you do that you call chiropractic? That would be fine, except a small faction believe that results are impossible to measure because they don't treat the obvious subjective symptoms of a patient's complaint. This philosophical disguise makes it easier to remain uninvolved and protect them from accountability. You want the right to do whatever it is you do, without having to scientifically prove you do anything, because you don't treat anything that is measurable! Perfect. In any other endeavor, this is called a scam.

If you don't treat symptoms, then you have an obligation to improve (and prove) better spinal biomechanics. If you treat symptoms, then you have an obligation at least to prove you've improved the patient's subjective complaints by whatever means you use.

Let's recap: We can't agree on philosophy because it's not relevant in the scientific 1990s. We can't agree on art because some techniques work better than others and non-force soft tissue work really isn't chiropractic. We can't agree on science because you'll never be able to measurably prove chiropractic adjustments improve nervous system function. We can't agree on results because the purpose of care isn't to treat symptoms.

It's amazing chiropractic has survived as long as it has considering this lack of consensus. The only thing everyone seems able to agree on is how to spell chiropractic!

Like it or not, in the context of "science-as-hero" that the public has come to respect, science is probably the only hope for unification (and acceptance) of chiropractic. It is the only commodity that the public and the dominant health care establishment will embrace. It is the closest common point that can join all the factions within chiropractic.

Sadly, this research can't come from chiropractic! Chiropractic research by chiropractors appears suspect and is often discounted by the medical community. Plus, few in chiropractic know the protocol and peer review process necessary for objective research to be considered valid. Countless projects within chiropractic "proving" its efficacy are flawed by ignoring this fundamental reality.

"But I get sick people well," proclaims the chiropractor proudly. "I don't need proof it works." Congratulations. But with the prevailing attitude of Scientism, that's not good enough. Arguably, your "results" could simply be the result of your caring tableside manner, producing a psychological healing, or that patients would have recovered on their own without your intervention anyway.

Ironically, much of the research needed to "prove" chiropractic already exists. The medical community has already proven what chiropractors treat (even if you don't treat symptoms!) and what normalizing spinal biomechanics does.

I think part of the problem is that many doctors wouldn't know what to do if they were totally accepted and didn't have to fight anymore. Part of the appeal of being the underdog is that every challenge, every delayed telephone call from the MRI facility, every payment-withholding tactic from an insurance company can be interpreted through this us/them, right/wrong filter.

The problem is, all too many chiropractors wouldn't know how to act if they were no longer the victim! ■

ARE CHEESEBURGERS HAMBURGERS?

When the very first hamburger was invented, the public was elated that they had an alternative to the sandwich, frankfurter, and the other fast food products of the day. A new generation of consumers flocked to retail outlets that served this new culinary delight.

The hamburger was attractive because it represented a new direction for fast food, contrasting as it did, not only in taste, but in being round instead of square. People who were tired of square sandwiches or had been unhappy with the mixed bag of Dagwood ingredients plastered between two sheets of bread, rejoiced. Now there was an alternative!

Hamburgers attracted a lot of attention in those early years. It was true that outspoken hamburger zealots proclaimed that hamburgers could solve any hunger problem. Some even suggested that the only food necessary for life itself was hamburgers! Some purveyors of hamburgers were thrown into jail for so closely imitating sandwiches, misleading the public with round buns instead of square, flat sheets. Fortunately, the outrage from the hamburger consuming public and the willingness of hamburger supporters to bail their leaders out of jail, led to legislation protecting the rights of the public to an unhampered supply of their beloved hamburgers. The only provision was that hamburger providers couldn't make sandwiches. Condiments were limited to ketchup and mustard. No luncheon meat specials, no submarine sandwiches, and definitely no grilled cheese on white!

Hamburger stands survived by offering a much needed alternative to sandwiches, and quietly educating their customers about the value of a "hamburger lifestyle." Because of economic competition, misunderstandings, and a bias against hamburgers, sandwich makers banded together to eliminate hamburgers from the fast food industry. A Committee On Cookery was established and secretly began spreading rumors about hamburger makers and the effects of eating hamburgers. "Once you start eating hamburgers, you'll have to eat them for the rest of your life," started as a nasty rumor and became accepted as common knowledge by an unsuspecting public. "Hamburger flippers are poorly educated" and "eating hamburgers will cause constipation" were added to the myths circulating about these simple handheld ground beef treats. Finally, it became unethical for members of the American Sandwich Association (A.S.A.) to fraternize with individuals that prepared hamburgers.

Despite the organized efforts of the A.S.A., hamburgers *didn't* go away. In fact, the lies and unfair trade practices seemed to make hamburger providers even stronger. Powerful word-of-mouth advertising from delighted customers attracted interest and a quiet, "hamburger underground" emerged. Often entire families would show up for lunch or dinner. Huge hamburger outlets thrived, some having to build airstrips and hotels nearby to handle the demand for their special brand of nourishment.

But when hamburger makers got together at their annual conventions, those unhappy with the slow progress and acceptance of hamburgers began to voice their frustration. "Because hamburgers are just as effective, perhaps more effective than sandwiches, in overcoming hunger pains, we should be treated as equals to sandwich outlet operators," they crusaded. "We want sandwich equality!" they demanded.

Those frustrated with the pace of acceptance decided to take matters into their own hands. "Let's be more like sandwiches, so it will be easier for the public to accept us!"

It started as an experiment. First it was the addition of lettuce to the simple hamburger. Many hamburger customers, especially new ones, seemed to like the color, taste, and texture of the new burger.

While this small, seemingly insignificant change to the hamburger was dismissed or ignored by many hamburger outlet operators, no one could overlook the next development in hamburger "progress" and hamburger "acceptance" . . . cheese.

Every hamburger chef had been warned about the cheeseburger. In fact, the early hamburger pioneers specifically wrote about the temptation to add cheese, pickles, onions, and even bacon to the simple and elegant hamburger. "You'll mix up the dining public and lose the unique factor that make hamburgers, hamburgers," decried the earliest hamburger visionaries. "The very survival and integrity of the hamburger profession is at stake," crusaded the pioneers. "Your legal right to even exist is solely dependent on your distinctness and unique contribution to feeding a hungry world."

"But the public likes the special sauce and the convenience of getting a sandwich-like hamburger," argued the innovators. "Besides, scientific research proves that these additional ingredients improve the taste and digestion of hamburgers. Anyway, a cheeseburger is still a hamburger."

The hamburger industry divided into two factions. The hamburger side formed its own lobbying groups and industrial standards committees. The cheeseburger faction formed a different organization with its own committees and cheeseburger standards. Hamburger chefs everywhere had to choose sides.

The sandwich makers delighted at this internal conflict. They had seen the results of this type of disagreement years earlier among the submarine sandwich industry. Apparently the submarine sandwich makers had fought about the "purity" of their sandwiches, but ultimately sold out and were absorbed by the larger, more accepted mainstream sandwich community.

With the encouragement and financial help of the huge cheese and pickle industries, the cheeseburger faction increased in size and political clout. Since more money could be charged for cheeseburgers, bacon cheeseburgers, and double deluxe cheeseburgers, the incomes of the cheeseburger providers increased. Some cheeseburger providers learned they could increase their profits still further by emphasizing the less costly ingredients of their cheese and pickles. Soon, the amount and quality of the meat in an increasing number of cheeseburgers diminished. Advertising slogans and jingles praised the special sauces and other hamburger dressings. To the alarm of many, some of the most "modern" outlets even started calling their cheeseburgers "sandwiches." More and more customers were left with the impression that the hamburger toppings were actually more important than the hamburger!

Being so much like a sandwich, an increasing number of cheeseburger makers jumped at the chance to charge the same for their burgers as the higher-priced sandwiches. After years of lobbying, cheeseburger equality was finally achieved. As the differences between sandwiches and cheeseburgers blurred, the number of cheeseburger providers increased, leaving the strict hamburger contingency a vocal, but politically weak minority in the burger community.

The cheeseburger faction was feeling pretty smug about the time an interesting economic phenomenon occurred. Cost containment organizations emerged, first excluding burger providers, then admitting, but severely limiting the reimbursement on the number of burgers eaten. With the overhead costs associated with the storage and handling of countless hamburger toppings, the cheeseburger providers were the first to feel the pinch. With the focus on the toppings and reliance on third party payers, many cheeseburger chefs were suddenly at a disadvantage. Some had forgotten the value and virtues of the simple hamburger. Others were unsure whether the public would buy a simple unencumbered burger!

Ironically it wasn't the difference between cheeseburgers and hamburgers that ultimately separated the winners from the losers. Few members of the general public were even interested in the petty squabbling. It was when the sandwich makers started making hamburgers that things got rough!

"Get your hamburgers from the accepted experts in sandwich science!" screamed the advertisements. "Now get immediate relief of your hunger pangs from the makers of sandwiches that you've trusted since you were born!" smirked the TV commercials. "The best just got better!" said a leading sandwich distributor. "Why settle for just hamburgers when you can get everything you need at one convenient location?"

The moral of the story? A house divided cannot stand. The integrity and future of chiropractic is made more secure by being separate, distinct, and unique. The more we try to be like the "big dog," the less patients will have a reason to seek us out. Which would you prefer, to be liked or to be respected? Circumstances may force you to make a choice. I hope it's the right one. ■

ADDITIONAL RESOURCES

I credit much of my interest in reading and writing to my parents, who opted not to have a television in our house until I was well into the sixth grade. Instead, I have fond memories of Tuesday nights when we'd all go to the public library. We would each bring a stack of books home and dive in. All you could hear was the clock ticking as all of us had our noses buried in a book. I still do a lot of reading. Here is a list of some of the titles that inspired some of the chapters in this volume.

Brain Sell, Intellectual Strategies For Making The Sale by John Cantwell Kiley, M.D., Ph.D. I liked the way the author made strong points about keeping promises to ourselves and the importance of not necessarily telling customers (patients) what they want to hear. Short, practical and especially valuable, even if you're not an analytical like me!

Close To The Customer, by James H. Donnelly, Jr. This has twenty five down-to-earth suggestions for improving customer (patient) service and exceeding expectations. While it's aimed at the mainstream business community, there are a lot of ideas that apply to a chiropractic setting. In particular, idea number nine, which explores what happens when patients have a less than optimum experience in your office.

Everything You've Heard Is Wrong, by Tony Campolo. This one, and Larry Burkett's, *Business By The Book* are excellent contemporary validation for the importance of sticking to your value system when doing business in the 1990s. Tony doesn't pull any punches. His in-your-face reality check can serve as a much needed kick in the pants, if you still don't know why you're on this planet!

Influence, The New Psychology of Modern Persuasion by Robert B. Cialdini, Ph.D. My friend Steve Perman, D.C. put this book in front of me, and what an eye-opener. The chapter on Commitment and Consistency should be required reading for anyone interested in improving patient compliance. You'll probably blush as I did as I discovered how direct marketers, infomercial producers, and effective sales people get us to do things we might not ordinarily do.

Intellectual Capital, How To Build It, Enhance It, Use It, by William J. Hudson. Don't be put off by the title! This one affirms why the "idea" of chiropractic is an especially valuable currency in this day and age. We don't live in a zero sum economy! Our success doesn't mean someone else has to lose. Get some great ideas that will help you respond to the future with a better attitude.

230

Patient Satisfaction Pays, Quality Service For Practice Success, by Brown, Nelson, Bronkesh, and Wood. I wish I'd written this one. While their principles apply to all types of health care providers, there's plenty of valuable information you can put to use in your office. They echo my opinion, that some of the most important components of satisfaction, compliance, and referrals have little to do with the actual procedure or the outcome for which a patient consults your office. It has a textbook tone, but it's full of great ideas and observations.

Raving Fans, by Ken Blanchard and Sheldon Bowles. Ken entered our consciousness years ago with his *One Minute Manager* series. This, his latest book, uses a contemporary parable to demonstrate ways of creating delighted, loyal patients. Devour it in one evening when everyone else is watching the tube.

Stewardship, Choosing Service Over Self-Interest, by Peter Block. This book articulates a management style I've been trying to perfect in my business. Say goodbye to paternal, authoritarian control, and benefit from a practice that actually treats staff members as partners. Most of this goes 180 degrees counter to the typical practice management approach, but explore new ways to organize your office.

The Only Thing That Matters, by Karl Albrecht. Karl has crystallized and focused his approach to improving customer service in his latest book. One of his best ideas is to have staff members list all of their major job functions, and next to each one, list what the patient expects, then brainstorm in a third column ways to *exceed* a patient's expectations. Great staff meeting exercise!

The Paradox of Success, When Winning at Work Means Losing at Life, by John R. O'Neil. In the *Star Wars* trilogy we were introduced to the "dark side" of the force. Mr. O'Neil calls it the "shadow." With the exception of expensive therapists, there are few places that leaders, such as chiropractors, can look for guidance in bringing balance, renewal, and sensitivity to the office. If you throw a fit when you're not treated like an important person, read this book immediately!

What Do Your Customers Really Want? by John F. Lytle. More customer (patient) service insights. Find out why most patient surveys are a waste of time and what to do instead. Tap into some of the many unexpressed patient needs and discover new ways to enhance the word of mouth process.

Your Own Worst Enemy, Understanding The Paradox Of Self-Defeating Behavior, by Steven Berglas, Ph.D. and Roy F. Baumeister, Ph.D. Have you ever seen someone "choke" at a critical moment in their performance? Have you ever wondered why especially successful people (Jimmy Swaggart, Gary Hart, Pete Rose, etc.) end up getting caught doing stupid things? Are you guilty of self-defeating behavior? Get some valuable insights into avoiding practice sabotage.

William D. Esteb, co-founder of Back Talk Systems, Inc., provides a variety of seminars, consulting services, and communication tools to enhance patient education. Call or write to receive a newsletter and a catalog of practice aids that reflect the patient-centered philosophy presented in this book. Mr. Esteb is available for speaking engagements on the topics presented in this and his two preceeding books, *A Patient's Point of View* and *My Report of Findings*. For more information contact:

William D. Esteb
Back Talk Systems, Inc.
2845 Ore Mill Drive, #4
Colorado Springs, CO 80904-3161
(719) 633-1105 or (800) 937-3113

232